NATURAL

ASTHMA

and

ALLERGY

MANAGEMENT

Natural Asthma and Allergy Management

Celeste White, M.S.

Keswick House
Redding, CA

The following names used in this volume are registered trademarks: Celtic Sea Saltô, Dr. Bronner's, Earth Rite, Inspirol, Intal, Knudsen's, Mother Earth's, Multi-Pure, Orange Mate, Primatene, Proventil, Scarmassage, Seldane, Shaklee, Shelton's, Similasan, Ventolin.

Neither the publisher nor the author has any personal, financial, or business relationship to the companies mentioned in this book.

ISBN 0-9653024-1-5

Library of Congress Catalog No. 96-95414

First Edition
2 4 6 8 10 9 7 5 3 1

Cover art by Diane Morley
Cover design by Candia Ludy and Diane Morley

Additional copies are available. For your convenience, order information is included in the back.

For Aunt Connie

I would like to thank the following nice people for their help, contributions, and/or support:

Frank Campanale, L.Ac.
Edwin Stewart, D.C.
Richard Hardie
Candia Ludy
Diane Morley
Julie Coburn
Patience Harvey
Susannah Hardaway
Tim Schoch

TABLE OF CONTENTS

INTRODUCTION i

CAUSES OF ASTHMA AND ALLERGIES 1

CHINESE MEDICINE 9

WESTERN HERBAL MEDICINE 22

MIND/BODY MEDICINE 30

HOMEOPATHY 38

ENVIRONMENTAL FACTORS 47

EATING HABITS 60

CHIROPRACTIC AND OSTEOPATHY 73

BREATHING AND EXERCISE 80

MISCELLANEOUS CONSIDERATIONS 86

APPENDIX A

    ACUPRESSURE POINTS 99

APPENDIX B

    RESOURCES 101

APPENDIX C

    SUMMARY OF TREATMENTS 105

INDEX 110

¤   ¤   ¤

As patients themselves begin to understand their bodies in this new way, they…may begin to realize the extent to which the body that they present to medicine for diagnosis and treatment is a body of meaningful experience, a body of significant intelligence, inherently informed about itself; a body the very nature of which can be profoundly changed by virtue of each patient's sensitivity and embodied awareness, and his/her own skillfulness in articulating the body's carried meanings.

— David Michael Levin, PhD,
from "Meaning and the History of the Body:
Toward a Postmodern Medicine"

¤   ¤   ¤

Introduction

Asthma is on the rise, both in the numbers of people who are experiencing symptoms, and in its virulence and lethality. Urban areas in particular have seen a near explosion in the incidence of asthma, but the increase is occurring all over the globe, in all kinds of locations. If you're reading this book, you are undoubtedly one of the 10 million people in America who suffer from asthma— or you know and love someone who does. Perhaps you tried the best that modern allopathic medicine has to offer, like I did; but you're still suffering. You may be experiencing lots of unpleasant side-effects from your medication, and you're quite likely frightened, too: that you'll get worse, that you'll end up in the hospital, that you might even die.

Introduction

Those of you who have asthmatic children or partners know how scary this condition can be from the outside. You listen to them wheeze, feeling helpless and perhaps a little short of breath yourself, in empathy. You don't know when they might have a life-threatening attack. And you fear it could come at any time, for who knows what reason. In fact, I recently read a book by a man who felt that he had to live within fifteen or twenty minutes of an emergency room because of his asthma. Perhaps you or your family exists in a similar predicament. This is the bad news.

The good news? It doesn't necessarily have to be this way. In my personal experience, and the experience of countless others, asthma is very manageable. And you don't have to take a lot of medication to do this. I myself have gone from using my inhaler four times a day to four times a year (in a bad year!). I take no asthma medication and haven't, for five years. I've managed to stay out of the hospital completely (a good thing, since I don't have health insurance), and my overall health has improved dramatically. I treat my asthma and allergies with a combination of the modalities I discuss in this book: acupuncture, herbs, homeopathy, diet, mind/body techniques, and lifestyle changes.

In my opinion, anyone, no matter how severe their asthma, can achieve the same level of health that I have. Anyone! It takes commitment, effort, change, and perseverance, however. Asthma has a complex etiology and many people have spent years developing the conditions that lead to asthma. It's unlikely that you'll be able to clear it up in no time.

Unfortunately, our "magic bullet" mentality has made Americans poor candidates for enjoying the effectiveness of alternative treatments because of our impatience and insistence on instant results. Some people have experienced relief from asthma attacks in as short a time period as 30 seconds into an acupuncture treatment, but it's more probable that it will take several acupuncture treatments (as many as ten) before you notice a significant difference, if this is the treatment route that you choose. But if you stick with it, your chances for a distinct, even remarkable improvement, are excellent. Making the effort and investment is well worth it.

You will no doubt need to make several changes in your lifestyle, diet, etc., too. This can seem like a hassle at first, but if you feel the way I do—that being able to breathe is worth it—you can find a way to incorporate these changes into your life. After awhile, you hardly notice. And these changes will, in fact, lead to greater overall health, both mental and physical; they can help you to avoid other chronic health problems, such as arthritis, colon problems, heart disease, etc.

I am including allergies in this discussion because asthma and allergies are often integrally related, though sometimes people who suffer from one do not experience the other. However, what works for asthma often works for allergies. And if you do have to deal with both, clearing up one will help to clear up the other.

In addition, for those of you who are interested, I'm including some technical discussion on the ways in which alternative healing methods work on the biophysical and biochemical levels. For those of you who don't want or need to know about this type of thing, you can skip over these sections and still make full use of the practical information provided.

A chronic illness such as asthma can make you feel vulnerable—even like an invalid. It can rob you of obtaining the full pleasure that life has to offer and it can diminish your entire experience. But it doesn't have to be this way. In my last book, I quoted from RITUALS OF HEALING, by Achterberg, Dossey, and Kolkmeier, and I would like to repeat what these wise healers have to say in this context as well: "Illness and the opportunity it presents people to engage consciously and actively in a journey towards wholeness can be one of the most transformative experiences that life offers."

This has been my experience. If you are currently burdened with a chronic illness such as asthma, I hope that it will be yours, too.

CAUSES OF ASTHMA AND ALLERGIES

Asthma occurs when our bodies respond to allergens by producing histamine, a chemical substance that causes the lung tissue to swell and the smooth muscle of our lungs to constrict. When this happens, the diameter of our bronchioles (the branching tubular structures through which our lungs draw air) shrinks, obstructing easy airflow. This is when we start wheezing and our lungs start whistling and we feel like an eight-hundred-pound gorilla is standing on our chests. A highly unpleasant, if not terrifying sensation.

Predispositions and triggers

Medical science characterizes asthma as a poorly understood disease. No one knows why some people react to normally harmless substances such as pollen or animal dander by producing histamine (which also produces other allergic symptoms besides asthma), and others don't. A good friend of mine who is a trauma surgeon feels it is a result of an immune system that is too tightly wound, while those who are susceptible to chronic infections or cancer have an immune system that is too lackadaisical and unresponsive. This seems to me to be an accurate observation; I feel, in addition, that those who suffer from asthma and allergies have a genetic predisposition to the illness.

Our bodies have a limited number of symptoms that they can express. They can throw up, run fevers, get rashes and bumps, turn different colors, bloat and distend, bleed, discharge fluids, etc., etc., but all of those symptoms don't add up to the number of diseases that we can possibly come down with. There are far more diseases and syndromes than there are symptoms; therefore, lots of dissimilar diseases produce similar symptoms. Lyme's disease can mimic arthritis, chest infections can be caused by either viruses or bacteria, and some people mistake indigestion for a heart attack. This is why diagnosis can be so tricky. In my opinion, people who have asthma are genetically predisposed to respond to certain bodily assaults in the form of histamine production. Other people might develop cancer, diabetes, depression, or ulcers.

But a predisposition is only that: a predisposition. Triggers also play a role in creating the syndrome. Asthma can have many triggers. For some people, it's oak pollen, for some, it's dry-cleaning fumes, for others, it's cat dander. Many people don't have asthma as a child but develop it as an adult. Some people have it as a child but outgrow it when they get older. Some people have it as a child, it goes away for awhile, and then it comes back. Triggers are not the same thing as causes, however. The cause, I believe, goes far deeper.

Pollution

Asthma has been around for a long time; probably as long as there have been humans. But no one is disputing the fact that asthma is on a precipitous increase. And it's clear to every statistician and researcher that urban areas are experiencing the worst problems. Studies undertaken to determine whether the cause is air pollution have been deemed inconclusive by some researchers, but other health watchers feel that the evidence is unambiguous: the increase in asthma is directly related to the increased amounts of certain chemicals in our air.

Even so, I question just how many different pollutants were considered in the studies and whether the synergistic interaction between different kinds of pollutants were taken in consideration. In my view, it is not just air pollution that may prove to be the culprit. Pollutants ingested from our highly chemically treated water and food could also be part of the problem, as could our highly disruptive electromagnetic environment. Electromagnetic fields have been shown in countless studies to have physiologic effects on living organisms.

It's no coincidence that Romania, one of the most horribly polluted countries on the planet, also has some of the highest number of severe asthma cases on the planet. In Romania, the only thing that can often be done for asthmatic children is to keep them in caves. So, it seems quite clear to me that toxins ingested, inhaled or absorbed comprise a significant factor in the cause of asthma.

<u>Stress</u>

I also feel that stress is a significant factor in the development of chronic health problems. Stress and depression have been shown in numerous studies to have pronounced and negative effects on the activity and effectiveness of natural killer cells, which search out and destroy tumorous or infected cells in our bodies. Stress and depression have also been shown to decrease the levels and activity of immunoglobulins and interferon, both important molecular tools of a healthy immune response. Asthma and allergies are definitely malfunctions of the immune system.

Moreover, studies have shown that poor children who live in urban areas are some of the most vulnerable to asthma; given the stress that their living conditions can inflict, it's no wonder that these children are suffering from asthma. It's also true that most asthmatics experience stress-related attacks and that the stress of the asthma episode itself can often accelerate and worsen symptoms. Stress is a constant, unremitting part of modern life in just about every part of the globe, whether it derives from famine, ethnic and/or religious clashes, traffic, insecure employment, breakdown of communities and families, overcrowding, etc., etc. Stress is widespread and pervasive.

Inhalers

Another possible factor in the rise in asthma could be related to one of the most widely used remedies for asthma. My personal experience, though M.D.'s might disagree with me on this, is that long term use of inhalers can cause long term rebound effects. A study published in the British medical journal, *The Lancet*, did show, however, that infrequent use of albuterol inhalers proved more effective than regular use in reducing the symptoms of an asthma attack. And these days, even most allergists and pulmonologists will tell you that using noncorticosteroid inhalers for emergencies only is better than using them several times a day. (Some people's asthma, though, is so bad that they don't feel they have much choice.)

The prevailing medical opinion is that struggling for breath causes lesions to form on the lungs and that these lesions can lead to more frequent or severe episodes. This is why allopathic practitioners feel it's best to use your inhaler the minute you find yourself gasping for air. But I feel that my asthma worsened after several years of using an albuterol inhaler once a day. (When I tried a corticosteroid inhaler, it produced such intensely unacceptable side-effects that I stopped using it after a week.) I have also found that if I "work through" an attack by using breathing techniques, acupressure points, and homeopathic tablets—rather than automatically reaching for my inhaler—I do better over time and I have fewer episodes in general. The lesion theory doesn't seem to bear out in my personal experience.

Drugs

Taking any kind of drug long term, whether for asthma or anything else, weakens organ function. Which organ is affected depends on which drug you're taking, but just about all pharmaceutical drugs have a negative effect on the liver, which is where toxins are processed. If toxins building up in the body are a problem for asthmatics, then it's clear that taking pharmaceutical drugs will weaken your condition over time. Many asthma drugs are hard on the heart, too. And since the heart is the organ that distributes oxygen throughout our bodies, as well as cleansing our tissues of carbon dioxide, it is also clear that anything we take that interferes with the optimum functioning of the heart is going to have a long term negative effect on our asthma.

The new corticosteroid inhalers are supposed to restrict their action to the lungs, but that was not my experience. I developed severe vertigo after I started using one of those inhalers; so, obviously more systems than my lungs were involved in this drug's effects. Actually, the fact that allopathic medicine would target only the lungs in its treatment of asthma reflects a profound lack of understanding of the illness in my view. The practice of treating organs all by themselves in isolation from the rest of the body is proving a short-sighted and ineffective healing strategy.

I would like to caution, however, that I don't recommend to anyone who is currently taking asthma medication that they simply quit cold turkey. Asthma is a complex and potentially lethal disease that requires the supervision of a professional health care provider in all but the mildest of cases. So, if you are currently taking medication but feel that you would like to stop, first engage the services of an acupuncturist, herbalist, homeopath, or other naturopathic healer in whom you have confidence to help you switch over.

In summary, after spending many years researching the disease and experimenting with my own health, I view the constellations of symptoms known as asthma and allergies in this way: They develop in genetically predisposed people after so many toxic assaults have occurred in or to the body that the disease is triggered. These assaults can even be accumulated in utero if, for example, the mother smokes, has a diet composed of highly processed foods, or works in a job where she is exposed to high levels of chemical toxins. Some people are more sensitive than others, and therefore, they can develop asthma from less of a stimulus than someone else who has a higher tolerance level. These toxins can come from any number of varied sources: food, water, air, drugs, electromagnetic environment, and emotional, sociological, or psychological factors. Most likely, several cumulative triggers will be involved. Treatment consists of 1) detoxifying your body so that it isn't overloaded; 2) desensitizing yourself so that you raise the threshold of what your body can handle; 3) avoiding those allergens you can, and 4) counteracting the effects of substances you can't avoid to which you are sensitive.

Any chronic or recurrent symptom that our bodies express is an urgent cry for our attention and an unambiguous sign that we need to change some part of our lives. To ignore this is to invite worsening of symptoms and even the development of more serious illnesses.

In the following chapters, I will describe and discuss many of the highly effective alternatives that exist for the treatment of asthma. (Again, feel free to skip the sections that discuss technical details of molecular mechanisms, etc., if all you're looking for is easily implemented, practical suggestions). Since no one's asthma is precisely the same or derives from exactly the same circumstances, it may take some experimenting on your part to find an approach that works best for you; you might find, like me, that a combination of approaches works best. Don't lose heart, however. According to the famous healer Edgar Cayce, no disease is untreatable or incurable. If I can manage my asthma successfully, so can you.

CHINESE MEDICINE

By the summer of 1991, I had tried various pharmaceutical drugs, all without success: Theophylline, Proventil (both pills and inhaler), Ventolin, Primatene, Intal, Seldane, and a number of over-the-counter antihistamines. Not only did none of these drugs improve my asthma for more than a few days, just about all of them gave me extremely unpleasant side-effects ranging from nausea, accelerated heart rate, an arrhythmic heart beat, vertigo, nervousness, dry mouth, insomnia, and drowsiness.

Unwilling to start taking steroids, which seemed to be the only allopathic option left at the time, I called up one of our local acupuncturists. I felt vastly relieved when the receptionist told me that asthma and allergies were definitely treatable by Chinese medicine, since steroids such as prednisone have even worse side-effects than those listed above. Three months after seeing this practitioner, I was taking no oral medication whatsoever and had weaned myself off my inhaler. Best of all, I was breathing more easily than I had in a long time.

General concepts

Chinese medicine is an ancient healing system that has been in continuous use for thousands of years. At the present time, over a quarter of the earth's population employs one or more of its therapies, which include primarily the use of acupuncture and Chinese herbs, but also diet, lifestyle, massage, and other techniques such as moxibustion. This discipline approaches disease from an entirely different perspective than Western medicine. In Chinese medicine, the aim is to promote the healthy flow of qi (energy, or life force) that travels through the meridians of our bodies, to balance the yin and the yang of our systems, and to maintain healthy relationships between the five phases or elements of the body (metal, water, fire, earth, and wood).

In Chinese medicine, a symptom such as asthma is believed to be caused by an imbalance in any of these systems. It is understood that each individual with asthma might have a different set of causes for their symptoms. Chinese medical practitioners use their diagnostic systems to determine where blockages, excesses, and imbalances lie in the qi of each of the different organs and their meridians.

Organ systems are not evaluated separately, but in relation to one another. Organs are usually considered in pairs; often one organ is hypoactive, which causes another organ to be hyperactive, to compensate for the under-functioning one. Any one of the organ systems could be affecting the lungs: the spleen, kidneys, liver, heart, adrenal glands, sex organs, colon, etc. Chinese medical practitioners will treat both systems, not just the lungs. Often more than two systems will be involved; the practitioner will treat the two that seem to be most important and this can change over the course of treatment.

In my case, the problem with my lungs was linked most closely to the condition of my colon. A few years before my asthma returned, I had started drinking black tea every morning (coffee I had always avoided because it made my stomach hurt). For most people, this would not be a problem, but in my case, the tea dehydrated my colon, making my digestive system sluggish and inefficient. Taking care of my asthma involved improving my digestion by eliminating the tea, increasing the amount of water I drank, and increasing the proportion of fresh fruits and vegetables in my diet. However, dysfunctions in other organs systems, such as the kidneys or adrenal glands, can also lead to asthmatic symptoms.

Terms

When referring to and diagnosing dysfunction of an organ or system, a Chinese practitioner will refer to properties such as cold, heat, dampness, dryness, and wind. For example, heat was rising from my colon into my lungs. These simple terms may sound quaint and poetic to Westerners, and therefore, unscientific, but the fact is, these are descriptive terms in just the same way as allopathic medical terms are, such as suppurating, distended, jaundiced, etc. Both sets of vocabulary possess meaning for the practitioner in the context of the healing method. Simply because a term sounds more technical does not mean it is more accurate or helpful.

Seasonality

The concept of the Five Elements and the properties that might affect or afflict them also introduces the concept of seasonality into Chinese medical treatments. Allopathic treatments for asthma prescribe the same substance—say, theophylline or Intal—year round because they are only addressing symptomatic problems of the lungs, which, according to Western medicine, do not change over time, necessarily, nor by season. But a patient diagnosed by a Chinese practitioner as having heat in the lungs, for example, would get a different herb combination in the summer than he or she would in the winter. In the summer, the weather is hot and herbs that contain heat can exacerbate the condition; the "hot" herbs could be used safely in the winter, however, and might even be superior.

Herbal treatments

Western medical researchers are often unwilling to endorse or even believe in the effectiveness of herbal treatments because they believe that there is only one "active ingredient" in a medicine. Opponents to herbal medicine also point out that concentrations of active substances can vary widely from plant to plant so that it is difficult to know just how much of a pharmacologically active chemical a person is actually taking.

However, the belief in the superiority of a single active ingredient is just that: a belief. It is easier for researchers to design experiments to test the efficacy of one single ingredient, easier to write up convincing grant proposals (especially for pharmaceutical companies who want to manufacture this single active ingredient), and much easier to satisfy the protocols of the FDA in approving new drugs. No one will argue that active substances, when mixed or taken together, have synergistic effects on one another. This is why it is important that your physician and pharmacist be aware of all drugs that you are currently taking. Certain combinations can be harmful or even deadly, such as Seldane and erythromycin. But there is no evidence whatsoever to suggest that a single active ingredient is superior to a well-balanced blend of ingredients for any particular ailment. In fact, in HIV research, medical workers are finding that what they call a "cocktail" of different pharmaceuticals is more effective in staving off the symptoms of AIDS than is one single drug.

Chinese herb combinations are designed from thousands of years of observation and experimentation with individual patients. They are intended to balance all aspects of the problem from which the person is suffering and they are combined to have the least number of side-effects. Many foods, for example, possess carcinogenic agents in them, but the same food will contain anti-carcinogenic substances that cancel out this affect. Ma-huang, also known as ephedra, is an herb commonly prescribed in combinations for asthmatic patients. But ma-huang that is not balanced with other herbs can have a negative stimulative effect on the heart, just like much of the asthma medicine on the market. In the Minor Blue Dragon decoction, ma-huang is blended with ginger, cinnamon, peony, licorice, and several other herbs in order to ensure that the heart is not adversely affected while helping to open up the bronchioles in the lung.

It is true that dosages of active substances might vary from plant to plant and herb mixture to herb mixture. But the fact that, in general, dosages from herbs are significantly less than what is found in a drug, in addition to the fact that many herbal treatments are blends, makes this objection less valid, in my opinion. On the other hand, this brings up a good argument for not prescribing your own herbs, unless the herb is extremely benign. Particularly when dealing with an illness as potentially life-threatening as asthma, it makes good medical sense to see a professional herbalist rather than try to self-medicate.

Environment of the body

Chinese medicine is far more interested in optimizing the total environment of the body in treating disease than it is in addressing or suppressing one set of symptoms. The combination of acupuncture, herbs, diet, etc. is all designed to create a healthy body environment or state. The philosophy of this medicine is that disease cannot take root in a healthy, strong, well-balanced body. For this reason, relief obtained from these types of methods is often not as dramatic and quick as that obtained from a shot of adrenaline or a powerful drug. The development of a chronic illness has often taken many years, and therefore, it can take awhile to get the body back into balance and harmony so that the condition will subside on its own. Chinese medicine encourages the body to heal itself, while allopathic methods tend to insist that the body perform in a certain way.

Unfortunately, allopathic methods for asthma seem to have more short term success than long term. It's almost as if forcing the body to behave just sends the problems farther underground where they continue to foment. My current acupuncturist tells me, for example, that he frequently sees asthma develop when a child has a skin condition. Once medicine is given to suppress the hives or eczema, or whatever, then asthma ensues. What needs to happen instead is to address whatever imbalance is creating the symptom of the skin disorder.

What to expect

Most acupuncturists are also Chinese herbalists and many now also prescribe homeopathic treatments, as well as supplements. Some (more traditional) Chinese doctors have you take home a big wad of sticks, twigs, leaves, etc., where you boil them into a foul-smelling tea to drink.

This is undoubtedly the best way to obtain the most active ingredients from the plant, but I have personally never taken herbs this way. Other herbalists prescribe either tablets or freeze-dried herbal powders. I've primarily taken the powders, which are mixed with water and then drunk, three to four times a day. They seem to work quite effectively. They can range in taste from a pleasant cinnamon, gingery, or licorice flavor to a somewhat peculiar creamed corn taste to some really vile concoctions that remind me of old tires. Some of them can be extremely bitter, too. If they're really awful, you can see if the herbs come in tablets or capsules.

But myself, I don't mind taking even the bad-tasting ones if it means I can breathe. Sometimes I think that caring for asthma is easier than trying to manage something like heart disease, which you're often not aware of. Not being able to breathe is so immediate and insistent that it's impossible to ignore. And being able to breathe is an outstanding motivator. Most of the herbs for asthma, though, are tasty and nice.

The first visit to the acupuncturist will probably take an hour to an hour-and-a-half. Several diagnostic tests will be administered and your history taken. The doctor will take your pulse (all twelve of them), check out your tongue, note all your symptoms, determine your overall appearance and manner, certain likes and dislikes, and he or she might also make use of kinesiology, or muscle testing. Usually, you will have an acupuncture treatment afterwards and then the doctor will prescribe some herbs or other remedies for you to take. Many acupuncturists these days use disposable needles, so if you're concerned about HIV or hepatitis, you can request them or choose a doctor who uses them. Reusable needles, however, are autoclaved, and there isn't a virus alive or dormant (that we know of) that can withstand the thousands of degrees of temperature and pressure that they're subjected to in an autoclave. So, you don't really have to worry about this.

The acupuncture treatment

The treatment itself is overall a pleasant experience, though there are a couple of not-so-terrific aspects, too. The main one is that as soon as all the needles are set in my arms, elbows, wrists, and hands, and the doctor has left the room, my nose starts itching violently. That's the worst part. Sometimes when the needles go in, it feels like someone tapping you on the skin; sometimes (though much less frequently) you'll get a shock, one that might travel for an astonishing distance. It rarely hurts. It's certainly nothing like having blood drawn, with that big gauge needle. It's not even like a hypodermic syringe, which also requires a certain diameter to be able to deliver fluids. The acupuncture needles are extremely slender and once they're inserted, you can't even really feel them. Of course, some practitioners are gentler in their insertion technique than others.

Once the needles are inserted, endorphins start flowing throughout your entire body and your meridians start balancing, which is a lovely, subtle, euphoric feeling.

Sometimes you will have needles inserted on both the front and back sides of your body, sometimes just one. Some practitioners use electronic needles instead of traditional needles, and these aren't inserted; the acupuncture points are stimulated with an electric current. Some acupuncturists like to work exclusively on the patient's ear, which apparently has a mini meridional map that reflects the entire body. The treatment lasts anywhere from thirty to sixty minutes.

When it's over, you should sit quietly for a minute before getting off the table. Don't just leap up. Aerobic exercising afterwards is not a good idea, either. I generally have no problem driving afterwards; most people don't. If you do, however, you should make arrangements to have someone take you to and from your appointments.

Acupressure

Acupressure is an alternative to acupuncture, but my experience, and I think a lot of people's experience, is that the effects are milder and don't last as long. For those who have a phobia towards needles, however, it might be more appealing, and in some communities, it might be your only choice. In addition, acupressure is a good thing to learn for yourself, to help out in situations when your breathing tightens up. The basic treatment philosophy is the same for both acupuncture and acupressure, which is to clear energy blockages in the meridians. I've included a few points to try in Appendix A, for both asthma and hay fever.

Insurance considerations

Fortunately, more HMO's and health plans are beginning to recognize the efficacy of acupuncture and Chinese medicine, so they are starting to cover these types of treatments. If your plan does not cover them, however, you should seriously consider paying for them out of pocket. Though it may seem expensive, in the long run, it really isn't, especially when your health is in the balance. The year that I started seeing a Chinese medical practitioner, my husband and I were living on $12,000 a year (and I'm not talking about the 70's) and we didn't have health insurance. One unfortunate aspect of health insurance is that it makes us think we can't afford things we used to pay for out of pocket. Besides, if you add up all your deductible expenses, meds, lost days at work, etc., you might find that it is actually cheaper to pursue these alternatives.

Finding a practitioner

Usually you can find a Chinese medical doctor by looking under "Acupuncturists" in the yellow pages of your local phone book. If possible, you should select someone with the initials "L.Ac." after their name, as this indicates that they are a licensed acupuncturist, and a personal recommendation from someone you know and trust is always helpful. If you don't like the practitioner you choose on the first meeting, then try another one. But don't be put off if he or she suggests that you will need a course of treatments. They're not trying to rip you off; this is the way the healing method works: slowly, subtly, and over time. Of course, as with all health practitioners of any variety, whether allopathic or holistic, quality varies from individual to individual. Some Chinese medical doctors are better than others. This is why obtaining a recommendation can be very important.

If you experience no relief after following through the recommended number of treatments (often ten), then you can safely deduce that this method is not working for you. This would still not make the visits a waste of time, however, as acupuncture works on balancing all systems of the body. One nice side benefit for me in having regular acupuncture visits is that I often don't get the colds or flu that are circulating in my community. If I do, my symptoms are usually much milder than everyone else's.

Those who live in small, rural communities may have difficulty in finding a Chinese medical doctor in their town. In this case, traveling once a week or every two weeks to a metropolitan area in order to see an acupuncturist might be worth the trouble if your asthma is severe. Or, you might try getting together with other people in your community to see if you can recruit a practitioner. As a last resort, you might try purchasing a good book on acupressure and asking a family member to help you apply pressure at the proper points; or you could stimulate the points yourself. This would be a last resort, however, as the diagnostic skills as well as the herbal remedies that a Chinese medical doctor can provide are invaluable.

Allergies and Chinese medicine

Of course, allergies are also quite effectively treated by Chinese medicine. The acupuncture points and herbs will vary from those used to treat asthma (though some will overlap). Food and other allergies can be tested for by your practitioner, too. Acupuncture is extremely helpful for hay fever, rhinitis, headaches induced by allergies, and all other allergic symptoms. In addition, stimulating acupressure points can do a lot of good as well; check out Appendix A for some points to try.

These days, I take no asthma medication, anti-histamines a few weeks out of the year during the worst of the allergy season, and at most, I use my inhaler a few times a year for emergencies. My overall health is greatly improved, and in fact, even my state of mind is calmer and clearer. If not a miracle cure, Chinese medicine is, in my opinion, one of the most effective treatments for asthma available.

WESTERN HERBAL MEDICINE

Western herbal medicine has a long and illustrious history in the same way that Chinese Medicine does. Humans all over the planet have been using medicinal plants to treat their ailments since prehistoric times. Many drugs on the market today possess ingredients derived or copied from a plant substance, and in fact, much of the action of herbal medicine is similar to pharmaceutical medicine. When they are ingested or inhaled, certain biochemical constituents in the plant have particular effects on the biochemistry and physiology of animal systems. For example, one of the effects of garlic is to reduce platelet aggregation, which prevents blood clotting.

For many reasons, such as the fact that herbs cannot be patented nor tested according to current FDA standards and the fact that their effects are often subtle, they have gradually fallen out of use in modern times in the United States. Nevertheless, in the last ten years or so, partly due to the number of side-effects produced by pharmaceutical drugs, interest in herbal medicine has resurged rather remarkably.

Herbal practitioners

Though herbs can be extremely gentle, they can also be extremely powerful. Because of their potential potency, and the fact that certain herbs in certain combinations can have interactive and even harmful effects, I would recommend that you seek out a professional herbalist to treat your asthma and allergies, if this is the treatment method you choose. Herbology is a complex and artful science, and it takes experience and knowledge to be able to heal effectively and safely with herbs.

Western herbalists do not have a licensing system in the same way that acupuncturists do, so it would be wise to obtain recommendations before selecting a particular practitioner. An excellent resource to contact in looking for a practitioner in your area is The Flower Essence Society, a nonprofit referral, networking, and educational service (see Appendix B for their address, phone number, Web site, etc.) They maintain a computer data base of over 60,000 alternative practitioners, stores, and classes. In addition, most naturopaths are well-trained in herbal medicine (among other modalities), and in some states, naturopaths are now being licensed; so another resource to try is the American Association of Naturopathic Physicians, which provides referrals to accredited or licensed practitioners all over the country. Their address and phone number is also listed in Appendix B.

Herbal remedies

For those of you who are not suffering terribly from asthma and/or allergies, and you would just like a few benign herbal solutions that you can purchase and administer yourself, herbs that fall into the category of tonics can be very helpful. Tonics work by strengthening general systems of the body or by imparting more vitality to the body as a whole. Tonics can be taken on a regular basis, over time, without any negative consequences. In addition, herbs in the category of expectorants loosen and help to expel mucous secretions that can make breathing difficult, particularly if your asthma or sinus problems are exacerbated by a cold, flu, or respiratory infection. Expectorants can usually be taken with impunity, too. Some herbs, however, such as stimulants, have effects that make their indiscriminate use more problematic and should be taken only under supervision.

Another consideration to keep in mind is the form in which you obtain your herbal remedies. Teas are usually the freshest and most potent, but they are often the most hassle to prepare and take. Tinctures and good freeze-dried extracts are usually a nice compromise between freshness and convenience. Tablets and capsules are the most convenient, but they are the least potent.

Stinging nettle is an excellent tonic and it has a wonderful reputation for helping asthma and allergies, particularly symptoms such as sneezing, stuffy or runny nose, itchy eyes, etc. Dr. Andrew Weil, in his book, SPONTANEOUS HEALING, recommends obtaining a high quality freeze-dried extract and taking one to two capsules every two to four hours (see Appendix B for a mail-order source). He also recommends taking the supplement quercetin, which is obtained from buckwheat and citrus fruits. Its mode of action is to stabilize the membranes of cells which release histamine, so that not so much is released into your system. Quercetin is usually available in health food stores.

Red clover is a wonderfully effective tonic that cleanses the blood and is extremely helpful for asthma, hay fever, and eczema. It has no toxic effects and can be taken safely on a regular basis. Another benign tonic that is a good immune system builder is Siberian ginseng. It strengthens the adrenal glands, imbalances in which are often linked to asthma. Appendix B lists sources, or look for them at your health food store.

A German company named Heel makes a terrific nasal spray that is herbally based, and I use it often during allergy season. It's called Euphorbium, and not only is it wonderfully effective for clearing stopped-up nasal passages, it has no rebound effect and sometimes can also ease asthmatic symptoms. When you inhale the mist, some of the solution goes into your lungs as well as into your nose. See Appendix B for a mail order source.

Yerba santa and marshmallow, which improve digestion, are herbs worth trying in your asthma and allergy management. Poor digestion is often a contributing factor to asthma and allergies, as efficient elimination is necessary for getting rid of toxins. A healthy colon will make a noticeable difference.

Thyme, elecampane, and mullein, all expectorants and immune enhancers, are other herbs to consider in treating your asthma and allergies (check out Appendix B or your favorite health food store). A nice balm to put on your chest when you're having trouble breathing is to purchase essential oils of thyme, eucalyptus, rosemary, and ginger (available at your health food store). Mix together a half-ounce of almond oil and a half-ounce of grapeseed oil (also from the health food store) and then add 5 drops of the thyme, 6 drops of the eucalyptus, 10 drops of the rosemary, and 14 drops of the ginger. Mix it all up and smooth onto your chest.

Ginkgo, originally from China but now widely used in the West, is often helpful for asthma as it prevents the bronchioles in the lungs from constricting. It's beneficial for your brain as well, since it increases blood circulation to that organ. It is such a popular herb right now that obtaining it should be easy, at either your local health food store, or even in drug stores or grocery stores. You can also check Appendix B for mail-order sources of high quality ginkgo.

Astralagus is a Chinese herb, too, but its effectiveness in boosting immune function has made it popular in the West for all kinds of ailments. I took this herb during the beginning stages of my treatment for asthma and I think it was helpful. It not only helped my immune system, of which asthma and allergies are a malfunction, it gave me more energy. Astralagus is usually available at your favorite health food store; suppliers are also listed in Appendix B.

Ephedra, or ma-huang, is another Oriental herb that is now commonly sold in health food stores and used as an anti-asthmatic. In my opinion, however, it doesn't really fall into the benign herb category. Two of its constituents are ephedrine and pseudoephedrine, which behave as stimulants, negatively affecting the heart and worsening hypertensive conditions. In fact, it is much safer to take this herb in combination with other herbs, as in Chinese herbal preparations; and personally, I would take it only the under the supervision of a professional health practitioner. Taking Ephedra alone often induces an unpleasant jittery, speedy feeling, too.

Hyssop, alfalfa, lobelia, lungwort, Irish moss, and horehound are other herbs that are often used in the treatment of asthma. I haven't experienced or encountered dramatic results from the use any of these herbs, however, so I can't recommend one wholeheartedly over another. Differing responses of individuals to particular herbs or herb combinations is inevitable, given the fact that the causes and triggers of asthma are different from person to person and genetic composition differs from individual to individual. (I sometimes wonder if allopathic medicine's desire to find drugs that work for so many different people is partially responsible for the number of side-effects they produce.) As I've mentioned before, I feel the knowledge and skill of a professional practitioner will greatly improve your chances of obtaining success with herbal remedies, but if you don't have access to an herbalist or naturopath, you can try experimenting with freeze-dried extracts, capsules, or tinctures of these herbs to see if they provide you with relief. Follow the directions and dosages provided on the bottle or container. Try the herb for several weeks, unless you have a negative reaction, in which case, you should stop taking it immediately.

If you start mixing herbs, though, I do urge you to check with an herbalist to make sure the combinations are safe. And if you're taking more than one herb or herb combination, wait an hour between times when you ingest them. Also, taking herbs on an empty stomach and waiting a half-hour before eating improves their effectiveness. They are more readily absorbed on an empty stomach.

Flower essences

Another type of herbal approach to consider for managing asthma is the use of flower essences. These are extremely dilute solutions that contain liquid extracts of various flowers, whose properties help to relieve unhealthy emotional states and to promote healthy, harmonious emotional states. Different flower remedies address different emotions, such as jealousy, impatience, fear, or lack of confidence; or, on the positive side, generosity, patience, courage, or confidence, to name just a few. Since anxiety and other troublesome emotions have been associated with asthma (and other allergic symptoms), these remedies can prove extremely helpful in your overall treatment. You can seek out a flower essence practitioner (whose expertise and knowledge will improve your chances of using the correct remedies); or you can order the essences from either Flower Essence Services or Ellon USA. Flower Essence Services also provides educational and descriptive information about each flower and its properties; Ellon USA will send you a questionnaire to help you decide which remedies to order. Check Appendix B for their toll free numbers.

In summary, several herbal remedies exist that are beneficial for asthma and allergies. You will need to do some experimenting, either with or without the guidance of a practitioner, to find what works best for you. But taking herbs without employing any other strategies will probably be insufficient for successfully managing your asthma or allergies. Herbal medicine should be combined with other treatments and lifestyle changes, such as acupuncture, diet, environmental considerations, chiropractic manipulations, etc. As I stated earlier, asthma and allergies are not conditions that lend themselves well to magic bullet approaches.

MIND/BODY MEDICINE

It is well-documented that asthma is worsened by stress and over-excitement and that it responds well to mind-body techniques such as visualization, biofeedback, and relaxation techniques. For awhile, because the causes of asthma include psychosocial triggers and because asthma did respond well to these approaches, it was thought that asthma represented basically a psychosomatic condition or the neurotic response of a hypochondriac to unpleasant interactions. As our understanding of chronic illness increases in sophistication and the relationship between the mind and body becomes increasingly clear, however, this type of thinking has fallen out of vogue.

The fact is, our bodies respond metabolically and biochemically to our thoughts and emotions. Countless studies have demonstrated that depression lowers the activity of natural killer cells (immune cells which protect us from cancer and infection), that it decreases interferon production, and that it lowers production of certain types of immunoglobulins. On the other hand, experiencing uplifting emotions strengthens our immune systems: Harvard students who were shown videotapes of Mother Teresa going about her work possessed increased amounts of a particular type of antibody in their saliva, while the same students, when shown a film about Attila the Hun, had decreased levels of this antibody. Interestingly, repression of emotion has also been linked to weakened immune response and increased rates of cancer, whereas a healthy expression of emotion, including grief, enhances immune function and resistance to cancer.

At present, the mechanism by which our thoughts and feelings stimulate the production of chemicals known as neuropeptides, which then go on to affect our immune systems and physiology, is not known. My theory, published recently in the journal *Frontier Perspectives*, is that the electromagnetic fields and wavelengths generated by our thoughts and feelings affect the shape and therefore activity of the regulatory proteins that determine which genes are read and which aren't. Whether this mechanism is at work or whether it is some other mechanism, however, it is clear that thoughts and emotions generate the production of molecules that then affect the physiology of our bodies. A disease can certainly be in your head, but it's never all in your head. A complex, continual interchange is taking place between your body and your mind. It is literally impossible to separate the two.

Since asthma responds well to mind/body medicine, it makes sense to learn about the different techniques available and to incorporate them into your management strategy. These techniques can help in the short term to control an episode, and they can also be employed to improve your asthma over the long term.

<u>Visualization</u>

Visualization is a very simple technique that anyone can learn. Basically, you just need to experiment a little bit with conjuring up an image that is helpful to you. Two images have been particularly helpful to me: One is imagining the interior of my lungs as a vast, soaring cathedral full of open space and light. Another image, which comes, no doubt, from my background as a biologist, is to imagine a cross section of my lungs on a slide, stained green, with very large, well-dilated lacunae where the section of my bronchioles falls. But you can come up with any kind of an image at all. The main point is to imagine something that will open up the bronchioles and relax them. So, it's entirely possible that simply visualizing an extremely restful scene, such as drowsing on a blanket in a pool of sunshine, would be helpful to you. Or, you can use a memory of a particularly enjoyable time when you felt particularly fine and your breathing was unimpeded.

If one image isn't working, then try coming up with another one. Rely upon your intuition in this. The content of the image doesn't have to make logical sense. You are trying to communicate to your subconscious—the part of you that regulates your physiology—that you are relaxed and the smooth muscle lining your lungs should relax, too. While you are visualizing, try to stay as focused on the image as possible. Try not to let mental chatter impinge. When this happens, merely recognize the fact that it has happened, and return your awareness to the image you are creating.

Meditation/relaxation techniques

Relaxation techniques can also be quite helpful. One method is a simple type of meditation. Sit in a comfortable chair with your hands in your lap and close your eyes. Concentrate on the feeling in your hands or on a spot in the middle of your forehead. When you do this, you will most likely notice a tingling sensation. Maintain your focus on this sensation. Again, when mental chatter pipes up, acknowledge the fact, then return your focus to your hands or forehead. Some people like to concentrate on both areas simultaneously, and some people like to shift their awareness back and forth. Try different approaches to see what works best for you.

If you are unused to meditating, you will quite likely find this to be surprisingly difficult at first. Mental chatter can drivel on persistently, repeating old bits of conversations we've engaged in (or confabulating ones we wish we'd had!), dredging up annoying advertising jingles, replaying songs we listen to, making a list of things we need to do. You should attempt to meditate for at least twenty minutes at a stretch, though, even if you don't feel you're doing it very well. If you do this at least once, but preferably two or three times a day, every day, you'll find that it gets easier and easier. And you'll enjoy added benefits besides just improving your asthma. You will have more energy, feel more relaxed in general, lower your blood pressure, and find that your mind operates more clearly and efficiently.

Another classic relaxation technique involves progressively relaxing different parts of your body. Lie down on a bed or sofa, then start by directing your attention to your toes and feet, consciously relaxing the muscles in them. When they feel relaxed, move onto your ankles, calves, and shins...then onto your knees, your thighs ...your butt, hips, stomach, torso...your shoulders, arms, and hands...and finally, your neck, head and face. By the time you finish, you should be thoroughly relaxed from head to toe. Some people have difficulty consciously relaxing their muscles, so if this is a problem for you, a technique that often helps is to tense the muscles first, then let go.

As you do these types of relaxation techniques, you might begin to realize that most of the time you're holding yourself tense, almost as if bracing for a blow. I know I do. The more you can become aware of holding tension in your muscles and consciously letting it go, the more relaxed you will become in general, the less sore your muscles will be, and the more energy you'll have for activities you really want to pursue, once you're not expending so much holding your muscles in a tense posture. And it will improve your asthma overall, too. If you're diligent about this, your unconscious state will become a relaxed one.

Biofeedback

Biofeedback is a technologically sophisticated way of controlling normally unconscious bodily functions such as breathing, heart rate, and blood pressure. First, participants are taught a relaxation or visualization technique, although variations on this exist. Some practitioners teach the participant to operate a computer-generated video game with his or her brain waves. Second, electrodes are placed on the skin. The biofeedback device which is hooked up to the electrodes measures such properties as skin temperature, the electrical conductivity of the skin, brain wave activity, or heart rate. These measurements are translated into a series of beeps and flashes that the machine produces (or changes that occur in the activity of the video game), the rate of which varies depending upon the electromagnetic profile of the brain, heart rate, or skin temperature, etc., of the person hooked up to the machine.

By coupling the electronic feedback with relaxation or visualization techniques, the participant can gradually learn to achieve the desired effect (lower heart rate, blood pressure, etc.; one practitioner has even been able to affect blood sugar levels in patients with diabetes). Computers are also often used to interpret the results, since the biological systems involved are quite complex.

The effectiveness and beauty of this technique is the instant and quite tangible feedback. This can make learning considerably more efficient. Several sessions are required, however—as many as twenty to forty; but once the techniques have been assimilated, the benefits are often permanent. And again, this is a technique that can have far more extensive benefits than simply improving your asthma or allergies.

The advantages to these methods are that you are not putting any foreign substances whatsoever into your body, so you need not worry at all about side-effects. And if my theory concerning the connection between the electro-magnetic activity and the biochemistry of our bodies is correct, then these methods might ultimately be the most effective way to address chronic health problems at their root.

Given the overriding belief systems of our society, however, that such methods are not physically substantial enough to be very powerful, these methods often do not work for many people. As much as we would like to divorce the effects of our beliefs from the physiology of our bodies, in practice, this is just not the way things work. The Cartesian mind/body split is becoming less and less compatible with the experimental results that modern scientists and health practitioners are generating, and now it is quite clear that the effects of our beliefs, thoughts, and emotions are translated into the production of certain molecules. So, a negative belief about a process can hinder its effectiveness just as easily as an unshakable belief in a drug can guarantee the success of that drug (the placebo effect).

To this end, I would caution the reader about two different pitfalls: 1) If the treatment doesn't work for you, this does not necessarily mean that it is quackery. The electromagnetic activity of your mind could literally be blocking the process that needs to occur on a physiologic level. 2) Don't make a mind/body technique your principal way of tackling your health problems if you feel even the least bit skeptical about its effectiveness. This is just asking for trouble. I think that a combination of approaches might work best at first. Then, if you find noticeable relief from visualization, meditation, or biofeedback, concentrate on it. The key to managing your asthma and allergies successfully is finding something that works for you as an individual. These sets of symptoms don't respond well to the "one size fits all" approach to health care.

HOMEOPATHY

The mechanism of homeopathy is still a matter of heated debate. In fact, this mechanism has remained so mysterious and so fundamentally different from the way we think of healing as taking place, we have practically relegated it to the category of magic. Magic, of course, invites scientific scorn. But I must say, one of the most peculiar aspects of the modern scientific establishment, to me, is its willingness to declare that something *can't* work simply because scientists aren't insightful enough to figure out *how* it works. Lots of physical, experiential data exist to show that homeopathy works. But because science can't figure out how, according to its preconceived ideas, it has deemed the activity of homeopathic medicine to be nothing but placebo effect. (This dismissive attitude towards the placebo effect is itself strange, considering how powerful it is!)

When I was in college, a story circulating around biology circles purported that a group of prestigious scientists had undertaken a serious mathematical study and determined that bumblebees couldn't fly, according to the laws of physics. Fortunately for the bumblebees, they didn't need these good scientists to tell them how to do it, or to tell them they couldn't. They just flew. Even if this story is apocryphal, I think it is extremely instructive. We need to remember that our sciences are just our best efforts to understand and explain the laws of nature that we encounter. When we come up against something we can't understand or explain, it usually means that our understanding is wanting—not that the phenomenon itself is not taking place.

Background

Homeopathy was developed in the late 18th century by a well-known and respected German physician, Samuel Hahnemann. He noticed that ingesting certain substances when he was healthy would make him sick; and somehow (who knows how!) he got the idea that if large doses would cause illness in a well person, small doses of the same ingredient might elicit healing in an ill person. He then embarked upon a highly successful series of experiments with his patients, in which he determined that his hunch was correct. His results led to the development of his "Law of Similars" (also known as "like cures like"), which states that in order to cure an illness, one needs to take the very same substance that would cause the illness in high doses in a healthy person. In his attempts to find the least toxic concentrations of medications to administer, he experimented with more and more dilute solutions and found that potency increased with greater dilutions (Law of the Infinitesimal Dose).

Mode of action

Fortunately for the world of healing and medicine, Hahnemann's hunch led him down the right path, though it is likely that his reasoning was not entirely correct as to why these remedies work. More and more evidence is accruing, from labs in Europe and the United States, that the action of homeopathic medicine is electromagnetic, not biochemical. Indeed, it couldn't possibly be biochemical, since rarely is there even a single molecule of the original substance left in the dilution of a homeopathic remedy that is administered. An Italian physicist, Emilio Del Guidici, has proposed that water molecules form structures capable of storing electromagnetic signals that originate from their association with the "active" substance. The shaking (known as succussion) which is part of the remedy preparation is believed to maintain this electromagnetic imprinting of the water molecules, even when the original molecules are no longer present in the solution.

This explanation for the homeopathic activity of the dilutions is becoming increasingly borne out by experiments. What is not known is how this electromagnetic information is interpreted by the body to stimulate the healing response. It is believed that somehow the energy triggers self-healing responses on the part of the body. Recently I have come to wonder whether the focus on "like cures like" has perhaps made understanding the action of homeopathy more difficult. It is possible that, since the water molecules are imprinted by their association with the "active" substance, their imprint might, in fact, be complementary to the active substance, not like it. It might be this complementarity, or balancing, that actually stimulates the healing response.

Whether the electromagnetic information is complementary or somehow mimics the field of the original solute molecule, however, the electromagnetic energy contained in the water molecules could be communicated to the proper regulatory proteins for particular genes, affecting their shape and activity. As the specificity of the gene regulation process depends upon these proteins and their configurations, their activity (or cessation of activity) would set into play a cascade effect where certain genes are turned off, others turned on, and different enzymes and proteins are manufactured by the cell, initiating the observed self-healing process.

Whatever the actual mechanism, it has become rather difficult to ignore the studies that are piling up in journals all over the world that document the effectiveness of homeopathic medicine. In Germany, for example, many physicians are having more success curing pneumonia homeopathically than with antibiotics, to which bacteria are becoming rapidly resistant. If something works, I think we should give it a try. On a pragmatic level, who cares if we figure out why or how it works? And not only has homeopathy been shown to be quite effective, it is extremely gentle.

Classic vs. combination homeopathy

Nowadays, two different schools of homeopathy exist. There is the classic form of homeopathy where the practitioner attempts, through obtaining an extensive medical history, to identify the one substance the patient needs most. A homeopathic solution of this one substance is then administered. In the last couple of decades, however, a lot of research has gone into combination remedies for generic health problems. Homeopathic solutions for colds and flus, PMS, yeast infections, depression, fatigue, headaches, back ache—you name it—have now been developed by several companies. The theory is that the body will use the remedies it needs, while the unneeded ones will be sloughed off.

Classic homeopathy

I have not experienced the classic type of homeopathy, but I have received several positive reports from those who have, including a couple of friends who successfully treated their dog's skin condition by taking him to a homeopath. In fact, the repeated success of veterinary homeopathy is one argument against detractors' contentions that this discipline works by the placebo effect. In my opinion, homeopathy is a valid, viable choice of treatment for a wide variety of ailments, allergies and asthma included. So if you don't have access to an acupuncturist or you have a needle phobia, or the other types of treatment you've tried haven't brought relief, try a homeopathic practitioner. Along with other types of holistic health care providers, homeopaths are becoming more popular and available. Seek recommendations from friends or contact the Flower Essence Society (see Appendix B for more information) for a list of practitioners that includes homeopathic healers.

Combination remedies

I have, however, benefited considerably from using combination homeopathic remedies, and I can enthusiastically recommend three products that I've tried. Two are made by the company BioEnergetics, which hand-succussess all their remedies; their allergy drops and sinus drops are outstanding. I've cut back extensively on my need to use antihistamines by using their allergy drops. I used to take antihistamines six months out of the year; now it's only a few weeks, at the height of the pollen season—and we have one bad allergy season where I live. The sinus drops can also provide a lot of relief from hay fever symptoms, too. BHI (Biologic Homeopathic Industries) makes a simple and effective asthma tablet, which has pretty much replaced my inhaler for all but the most severe emergencies. I used to take them four times a day, but now I just take them as needed. Information on how to obtain these remedies can be found in Appendix B.

In addition, my current acupuncturist has been having me take a combination homeopathic remedy for the molds that normally inhabit our bodies. Our bodies are hosts to all sorts of microorganisms such as bacteria, viruses, protozoans, and fungi, most of which are either benign or beneficial. Apparently, however, in certain sensitive or out-of-balance individuals, these endemic mold populations can overrun their optimum concentration in the body, thereby sensitizing it to other triggers. This remedy does seem to help, for when I run out, I experience more wheezing and tightness in my chest.

The Healing Crisis

One other subject that I should mention in this discussion is that of the "healing crisis." Many homeopathic practitioners are of the opinion that true healing takes the patient backwards through all the illnesses and traumas they have experienced that have brought them to their current state of dis-ease. For this reason, patients who undergo a series of homeopathic treatments may find that they begin to experience symptoms from ailments that they suffered from in the past. This should not be cause for alarm. Once all the healing crises have been weathered, a healthy condition is restored.

Getting the most from your remedies

Given their subtlety and mode of action (probably electromagnetic), there are several precautions you can take to improve the effectiveness of your homeopathic remedies. First of all, if you are taking drops, place the drops underneath your tongue. There are lots of capillaries, etc., in this spot, so the absorption is increased. If you're taking tablets, place them under your tongue, too, and suck on them slowly. You can take more than one homeopathic remedy at a time, but you should refrain from eating, brushing your teeth, smoking, or drinking anything besides water fifteen minutes before and fifteen minutes after you take the remedy. (Although, the manufacturer at BioEnergetics informs me that his remedies are not so fragile.)

If you're taking drops, try not to touch the dropper to your teeth, lips, or anything else, to avoid contamination. If you're taking tablets, shake one into the top of the container and then drop the tablet into your palm from the cap. Don't reach into the bottle. Store remedies in a cool, dark, dry place; at the least, keep them out of direct sunlight and high heat (like leaving them in a locked car during the summer). Don't store them in any container besides the one they came in. Avoid using highly scented lotions, cosmetics, and lip balms, perfumes, colognes, and aromatic, volatile substances such as mint and camphor while you are taking homeopathic remedies, too. Aromatic compounds possess a lot of kinetic energy and they go charging around, engaging in a lot of jostling and elbowing on the molecular level; they can disrupt the electro-magnetic structure of the homeopathically imprinted water molecules.

If you're taking remedies on a plane trip, some practitioners recommend that you take your remedies out of your bag and carry them on you, to avoid having them x-rayed, though I've seen a sign at Heathrow airport that claims studies have determined x-rays do not harm homeopathic medicines. I don't know which is correct. I've had my remedies x-rayed and they seem to work fine afterwards. But theoretically, it seems that any kind of energy bombardment could have an effect, given the mode of action of these remedies.

As it is gentle, nontoxic, and effective, homeopathy is certainly worth investigating, at least as an adjunct to other types of care. And some people might find that it alone is sufficient to manage their symptoms, though, as I've mentioned, I think using several approaches is best. If nothing else, give some combination remedies a try and see if they help you. In my view, healing methods that make use of the biophysics of the body are rapidly on their way to becoming one of the most important therapies of the future, and homeopathy falls squarely into this category.

ENVIRONMENTAL FACTORS

Since triggers for asthma and allergies often involve substances that are inhaled, seeking or providing as stress-free an atmosphere as possible can be extremely helpful. In some cases, it's the most viable option. Dust mites, mold spores, animal dander, pollen, chemical irritants, smoke, and cosmetic products can all provoke an asthmatic or allergic episode. Some of these can be addressed by the choices you make in your home environment. Others are situations not under your control that you will have to avoid.

Dust mites

Many people are allergic to dust mites; in fact, it's probably one of the most common allergies. Unfortunately, mites are everywhere. They're almost like bacteria in that respect. They live on and in our bodies (in fact, there's one type that particularly likes to inhabit our eyebrows) and on just about every surface you can find.

They live in pillows, carpets, curtains, bedding, on the floor, on windowsills, and in the dust that settles on tables, counters, etc. It's impossible, obviously, to avoid them entirely, but if you're sensitive to them, it can help considerably to cut down on their numbers. This means keeping your home as dust-free as you reasonably can. Frequent dusting with a dampened cloth, vacuuming, and cleaning of bedding is important. (I would avoid using products that come out of a spray can, though, to dust, as this is just adding a volatile chemical to the air. A spray bottle filled with water is just as effective as any commercial dusting product. Oiling your furniture with a product that comes out of a squeeze bottle would be better, too, than using a product from a spray can.)

Mold

Mold spores are another ubiquitous allergen that can be difficult to avoid entirely; but you can cut down on your exposure to them, too. Unfortunately, if you live in an old house in a humid climate or a house with a basement that floods on a regular basis, you might have difficulty. Some people have actually had to move to a new house or a new location in the city they live in to get away from a troublesome mold. Though moving is a drastic solution, of course, if your asthma and allergies are severe and mold is the main culprit, finding an environment that is friendly to you can be well worth the trouble. It can cut down on a whole hosts of other measures that you might have to resort to.

If you are only marginally allergic to mold, keeping your house as dry and clean as possible (keeping the house warm enough in the cold months of the year and possibly installing a dehumidifier) can help. Also, it's a good idea—if you have a choice—to avoid wall-to-wall carpeting. Hard surfaces such as tile, hardwood or softwood floors, linoleum, etc., are best when it comes to living with asthma or allergies. Area rugs are not a big problem, normally, since they cover less square footage and are often made from wool or cotton; but most wall-to-wall carpeting, in addition to harboring molds and dust mites, outgases chemicals. Wool carpeting is far superior to synthetic carpet, for many reasons, but it is also more expensive. And, some people are allergic to wool. A company called Natürlich carries a lot of environmentally friendly floor coverings, so if you're interested, write for their catalog (see Appendix B).

Building materials

While I'm on the subject of floor coverings, I would like to mention a few other things about building materials. If you're building or buying a house, try to avoid interior particle board or chip board. These two products are often used to sheath a floor before installing wall-to-wall carpeting, and they are used in inexpensive cabinetry, too. They are loaded with glue (one reason why they're so darned heavy) and other volatile chemicals, and these take forever to outgas. Not only that, a lot of subcontractors use glue to adhere the floor sheathing to the subfloor; nails are far better, though they are more labor intensive and sometimes squeak after awhile (using the right kind of nails or screws will usually prevent this). Add a synthetic carpet to all of the above, and you've got a nice little chemical stew brewing in the air of your house that will last for years. Plywood is not as bad, but it still contains quite a bit of glue and it outgases formaldehyde, among other things. Using solid woods and tile is a better choice for floors. Tile or recycled wood flooring is probably the best choice of all since our forests are dwindling at a fairly alarming rate. And they're one of the most important factors in keeping our atmosphere healthy, oxygenated, and clean. For cabinets, consider using solid wood, perhaps with glass, or metal.

Chemicals

Avoiding chemical irritants can be much easier. Since inhaling the fumes from dry cleaning isn't a good idea, select clothing and other fabric items that don't need to be dry cleaned. It's also wise to avoid dry cleaning any of your bedding. If you do dry clean, air the item for several hours (or days) outdoors before sleeping with it on your bed or wearing it. Some dry cleaners are now switching to soap and water methods; call around. Use natural cleaning products in your home, too. These have become much easier to find now. Shaklee makes some effective and pleasant household cleaning products, as does Earth Rite. You can even find some of these products in mainstream grocery or variety stores; you can definitely find them through health food stores and food coops. Orange Mate makes a lovely air freshener that is nothing but resin extracted from the peels of oranges (they also have a lime and a lemon scented product).

Two books worth checking out are CLEAN AND GREEN by Annie Berthold-Bond, which gives recipes for making your own cleansers, and NONTOXIC, NATURAL, AND EARTHWISE, by Debra Lynn Dadd, which gives lots of good information on how and where to find earth- and people-friendly products; it also gives some recipes on how to make your own cleansers, cosmetics, etc.

Whatever you do, DO NOT use heavily scented detergents or fabric softeners. These can not only trigger asthma attacks, they can give you hideous headaches, AND they can cover you or your child's body with enormous hives. They are nasty products. And there's no reason to use them. Plenty of unscented, environmentally friendly and biodegradable detergents exist that leave your clothes quite clean and smelling fresh. If nothing else, try using Dr. Bronner's castile baby soap. Moreover, I don't really see any need to use fabric softeners, since it seems to me that most fabrics sold in the United States are quite soft these days. Gone are the days of having to use that old burlap bag for leisure wear.

Perfumes, colognes, and cosmetics

Perfumes, colognes, and aftershave lotions can also trigger attacks. If you bathe regularly, you really don't need them. If you have friends who love to slather themselves in perfume or cologne, you might have to ask them nicely if they wouldn't mind sparing your lungs and/ or sinuses when you're around them and foregoing the olfactory enhancement factor. For your own use, you should look for unscented or very lightly scented shampoos, conditioners, lotions, etc. Be sure to smell anything before you buy it. Some products advertise themselves as "natural" (a fairly meaningless term in today's world), but they reek with heavy scent. Even some products calling themselves "lightly scented" are too smelly for me.

Another place that you will often run into potentially troublesome fragrances are the scent strips that advertisers for colognes and perfumes insert in magazines. These can fill up your mailbox, car and house with asthma- or allergy-inducing fumes; touching them can give you trouble for hours. If you call the subscription department of most magazines and tell them you don't want these inserts, they'll make sure the magazines you receive won't have them.

Pay attention to your deodorant, too. Definitely avoid sprays and try alternatives to those heavily chemical-laden, healthy-sweat-preventing, potentially Alzheimer-inducing kinds. I use a salt crystal that's in a stick form and it works better than any other kind of deodorant I've ever used. It doesn't keep me from perspiring, which is good, because our bodies rid themselves of toxins through perspiration, but it's great for body-odor control. (Men: a very alluring and powerful pheromone is produced in men's underarm secretions; so don't undermine your sex appeal by nuking those pits.)

I myself don't wear cosmetics, ever since 9th grade when all my eyelashes fell out temporarily while I was aiming for the Twiggy look, and I don't miss them; but those who enjoy using cosmetics should look for ones that aren't loaded with chemicals and scents. Your local health food store will have a good selection. Appendix B also lists some mail order companies you can try.

<u>Pillows</u>

The type of pillow you use can be an important consideration with respect to asthma and allergies. Some people are so sensitive to dust mites that they do best sleeping with a pillow that is encased in a plastic or rubber cover, since dust mites love to burrow into pillows. On the other hand, some people are sensitive to plastic and rubber, so they might want to consider using an all cotton pillow, available from mail-order companies Garnet Hill, Seventh Generation, or Coming Home (see Appendix B). This is what I use, and it makes for a very comfy, clean-smelling pillow. If you're not allergic to down, then a down pillow is an option, but if you're even marginally allergic, I would avoid down in pillows, bedding, and clothing. Repeated exposure to a borderline allergen can turn it into a full-blown allergen. Use cotton substitutes, or possibly fiberfill, though some fiberfills outgas noxious chemicals. In minute quantities, to be sure, but it's worth trying to find alternatives. Quilted cotton, wool, and silk can be extremely warm and cozy, and there are lots of nice products made from these materials.

Animals

Allergies to animals can be a major problem. My allergy to cats is so violent and intense that I literally cannot spend more than a couple of hours in a house with a cat before my asthma gets so bad I have to leave to keep from suffocating. So far, I have not found anything that helps, neither the herbs I normally take, nor the homeopathic tablets I have for emergencies, nor taking antihistamines or asthma medication beforehand, nor using my inhaler. My current acupuncturist, who loves a challenge, is determined to get to the root of this problem and take care of it. I'm encouraging him enthusiastically, since the popularity of cats as a household pet has put a severe crimp in my social life. But so far, the only thing that I have found to work in this case is to not be around cats, or even occupy a space that has had a cat living there anytime in the last six months.

This extreme sensitivity might sound like a psycho-somatic reaction to anyone who has never suffered this way, but not long ago, I had an experience that demonstrated to me, at least, that hypochrondria was not the main operating factor in this situation. Last summer, my husband and I went to stay with his sister in her home in Colorado, a place I'd stayed many times in the past. This time, though, after I'd been in the house for a couple of hours, I started having a lot of trouble breathing.

Thinking it was perhaps the altitude or the pollen season or mold, I increased my herb intake and used my homeopathic tablets, and I started taking antihistamines, but in the middle of the night I awoke, unable to breathe. I used my asthma inhaler, which helped for about a half-hour, then I was just as bad as before. Rather than head immediately to the ER, I decided to try sleeping out in the car to see if that would help. By morning, I was lots better.

In the meantime, my husband had been doing some thinking. He said to me, "You know, the only time I've ever seen you react so violently to something is when you've been around cats. I wonder if the people who rented this house over the winter had a cat." The renters had been told that pets were not permitted in the house, but after we asked around the neighborhood, we found out that indeed, they had had a cat. It had been out of the house for a month, and the carpets had been cleaned and the walls painted. But the allergen, for people who are sensitive to it, is unbelievably virulent.

Apparently, it is an enzyme in cats' saliva, not the actual fur of the animal itself. Through licking and cleaning themselves, they spread the allergen over their fur, which then sheds. All cats possess this enzyme, whereas in the dog family, the presence or absence of an allergenic enzyme in the saliva is breed dependent. I am usually not too allergic to dogs, fortunately, though I've noticed golden retrievers give me more trouble than any other breed. Horses are another animal to which some people are allergic.

If anyone in your family is allergic and asthmatic, and you have an indoor pet, it's a painful reality that you or your family member might not improve as long as the pet is in the house. A lot of people are so attached to their pets that they are willing to suffer the symptoms, but you should be aware that your sensitivity could increase significantly the longer you're around the animal. If you or a loved one has bad asthma, then hanging onto a pet, however dear and beloved, is really a risky choice.

You will most likely not notice a big difference shortly after giving your pet away, however. Remember that the allergen can be active for up to six months, even after the house has been thoroughly cleaned. Homeopathic remedies specifically for animal dander exist on the market, so if your allergies are mild, they might give you some relief (BioAllers makes one, and it's usually available in health food stores). They haven't helped me, though. Also, there is apparently a product on the market that you can give to or smear onto an animal that supposedly will knock out the allergen, but I haven't heard from anyone that these methods work. You could try them, however.

Believe me, I love animals dearly (right now we have a house lizard), and I'm especially fond of dogs. I know firsthand how loving and supportive an animal friend can be. But seriously, you can be putting your health and even your life in serious jeopardy if you are severely allergic to an animal and you keep it in your home. You really should consider keeping your exposure to an absolute minimum.

Smoke

Smoke is another cause of asthma that is avoidable. If you have asthma or allergies and you smoke, you should quit. If someone in your home has asthma and you smoke, you should also quit. You're doing them a disservice if you don't. You should at least smoke only outside and keep the indoors smoke-free. Having a wood stove is a poor choice for heating, too, if you have asthma. No matter how good the stove is, some smoke will leak out, especially if it's windy outside.

Pollen

Pollen, on the other hand, is not avoidable. It's everywhere. Sometimes heading to the mountains or seashore can be helpful, if you have that kind of money and a lifestyle that allows you to do so. But most of us in the modern world don't have that option. We're stuck wherever we live, and the vast majority of climates have some sort of pollen season. If you're allergic to pollen, you'll have to find some kind of ongoing treatment to help you. Try any of the ones discussed in this book.

In addition, eating a teaspoon or two of local honey a day has helped many people acclimate to pollen in an area. Staying indoors during the worst of the pollen season can help, as can a filtered, air-conditioned environment. Air-cleaners are available, too; be sure to buy a good quality one. Some people (particularly in Eugene, Oregon, which is known in some circles as the Allergy Capital of the World) have found relief in wearing a dust or surgical mask during the worst of the allergy season. When I work outside in my garden during the spring, I wear one, and it makes a difference. Keeping your home relatively free from dust, which probably contains pollen grains as well, will help, too.

Working these changes into your life

Now, it might seem that all this switching over to natural cleaning products, avoiding dry cleaning, finding the right kind of pillow, choosing the right kind of building materials, etc., sounds like a gargantuan hassle. But if you just take one thing at a time and get into certain habits gradually, you'll barely even notice the change. (You don't have to do everything, either.) Next time you pick up cleaning products at the grocery store, buy ones that are not loaded with chemicals. Or join Co-op America. They publish the NATIONAL GREEN PAGES, a directory of companies that sell earth- and people-friendly products. In fact, take a few minutes right now to call up the mail-order companies listed in Appendix B and order their catalogs. Shopping by mail is even easier than shopping at the store.

The next time you go shopping for clothes, read the fabric content and cleaning directions on the label; select those with natural fibers and ones that don't require dry-cleaning. Get in the habit of washing new clothes before you wear them the first time, since most new clothes have been sprayed with formaldehyde (you know, that "new clothes" smell). And if you're building, just keep in mind what you're taking on by choosing certain types of materials over others. If you're already in a house that has lots of particle board, chip board, or wall-to-wall carpet, you can switch over gradually, or at least make sure that your home is well-ventilated.

As far as working outdoors is concerned, use as few pesticides as you possibly can. This might mean that your roses aren't as unblemished or your lawn as picture-perfect, and that some of those hideously ugly tomato bugs are going to get a few of your tomatoes. But in my opinion, these are small sacrifices compared to our health. Not only can a build-up of toxins in your body lead to allergies and asthma, they can lead to cancer as well.

One thing coping with my asthma has done for me is to realize how thoroughly saturated our entire environment is with chemicals, and just how unnecessary it is. There are natural substitutes for just about everything, and most of these products are actually superior to the chemical ones. The more we demand these products and the more we buy them, the cheaper and more available they will become. It's already happening; we just need to encourage manufacturers to continue in this positive direction. Their bottom line is, they're interested in making money; and if we show them they can make just as much or more without poisoning us or our environment, then they'll meet those needs and desires. And we'll all come out ahead.

EATING HABITS

As accumulation of toxins in the body comprises a significant factor in the expression of asthma and/or allergy symptoms, what we put into our bodies is of utmost importance. Developing and maintaining a good, healthy diet is probably one of the most important approaches to managing these ailments that you can take. Your diet should promote healthy elimination as well as avoid substances that can trigger or contribute to attacks. In addition, you should strive to include as many nutrients that foster a healthy immune system as possible.

Artificial ingredients

First and foremost, you should avoid artificial ingredients, additives, preservatives, and food colorings. Food colorings in particular have been linked to allergic and asthmatic reactions in sensitive people, and the sad fact is, unbelievable numbers of products in our society are laced with them, from candy, to processed food, to over-the-counter and pharmaceutical drugs, to cosmetics, shampoos and conditioners. Even so-called "natural" type products that you can find at health food stores and through catalogs often use them. Fortunately, you can find products that do not have food colorings, and usually these are at health food stores. But you need to get in the habit of reading the list of ingredients for everything you buy and consume. There is no compelling reason to use products that jeopardize your health just so they'll look more vividly colorful.

Artificial ingredients include BHA, BHT, benzoic acid, sulfur dioxide, and many others. If it sounds like a chemical, there are more than four syllables in the listed ingredient, or there are only capital letters in the ingredient, it is probably an artificial chemical. Some are used to preserve the color and "freshness" of meats such as hams, bacon, etc. Most sausages possess artificial preservatives and are probably best avoided; though there are some products (Shelton's is one brand in particular) that do not have artificial ingredients. Often local sausage makers don't use such substances, either.

Most commercial brands of cookies, crackers, and bread products are loaded with artificial ingredients. You can buy bread from your local baker, make your own (bread-making machines are very affordable these days and almost criminally easy to use), or buy breads that don't have preservatives. These breads you will need either to consume in a timely fashion or freeze, since mold will start growing on them sooner than breads that have been thoroughly saturated with chemicals. You can also find crackers and cookies at health food stores that are free from artificial ingredients. Or, you can make your own. Along with providing yourself and your loved ones healthier, tastier food, cooking or baking can be a really relaxing activity, which is also beneficial for asthma.

Eating organic

It is a good idea, too, to buy as many organically grown fruits and vegetables as possible, and if you can find organically grown meats and dairy products, these would be wise to substitute for food that is grown with pesticides, hormones, antibiotics, and then treated or processed with more chemicals. It's true that these products are more expensive than ones laced with artificial ingredients, but a single-minded pursuit of the bottom line has only lessened our quality of life in the long run. It's been more important to us as a society that we get the maximum amount of profit from our agricultural activities, so that reduced spoilage of goods and volume of sales have taken precedence over the health of the consumer.

This is short term thinking, however. It might be that you are paying less for a loaf of chemical-laden bread in the grocery store, but we are paying a very high cost in terms of medical care overall in this country. These chemicals not only exacerbate asthma, they contribute to cancer and other immune system problems as well. So, I think it is important that we use our dollar votes to support food that is really good for us in every way. And the more people do this, the cheaper these alternatives will become.

It is already being discovered that organic farming methods are just as cost-effective as nonorganic methods, once the switch has been made and the systems are in place. You might find that you enjoy growing some of your own fruits and vegetables, too.

Soft drinks

Commercial soft drinks are also best avoided, as basically, you might as well be swilling a beakerful of chemicals. In fact, this is what you're doing, with copious amounts of sugar thrown in. If you prefer artificial sweeteners, this is just another chemical that you are burdening your system with. (A note about artificial sweeteners: Scientists have not yet been able to figure out why, but they have found no evidence whatsoever to indicate that regular use of artificial sweeteners contributes to weight loss. In fact, the opposite appears to be true.) Knudsen's makes some delicious fruit spritzers that have no artificial ingredients in them at all nor do they contain added sugar; you can usually find them at the health food store, but some grocery stores and mini-marts carry them, too. In addition, natural cola syrups can be purchased from Home Health and The Heritage Store (see Appendix B) and then mixed with carbonated water or mineral water.

Sweets

Sugar and sweets have also been implicated in the worsening of asthma. Both allopathic and holistic healers stress that sugar and asthma don't make a good combination. Apparently, immoderate sugar consumption can weaken your kidneys and liver function, as well as deplete your adrenal glands. It's best to cut back on all types of sugar, but honey, maple and rice syrup, and beet sugar are better than white cane sugar. Using artificial sweeteners, however, is not a good strategy for avoiding sugar.

Fats and oils

Another food group well worth paying attention to is the type of fats and oils that you consume. By far and away the best types of oils to use are pure, cold-pressed, monounsaturated or polyunsaturated oils. Use olive oil, peanut oil, canola oil, sesame oil, corn oil, or walnut oil, but shun partially hydrogenated soybean oil (which is the oil of choice for most processed foods, including mayonnaise), cottonseed oil, palm oil, shortening and lard. Olive oil (particularly "virgin" or "extra virgin") is considered to be the queen of oils, and it has lots of health benefits besides helping you with your asthma and allergies. It helps maintain healthy ratios of "good" and "bad" cholesterol, for one thing. It is also good for your complexion and digestion.

Since safflower oil oxidizes so easily, creating harmful compounds, it might be best to avoid it; and corn oil and walnut oil are not considered to be as healthy as olive oil. But I think that as long as you are avoiding the partially hydrogenated and saturated oils mentioned above, you'll be okay. Butter is fine, too, in moderation. It is certainly much better for you than margarine, which is essentially a stick of chemicals. Be sure to purchase fresh oils and butter and don't keep them on hand for too long. Rancid oil is extremely unhealthy. And by the way, you should keep your fat intake to a minimum, for both your asthma and your general health.

Water

Of course, drinking lots and lots of water is essential to managing asthma and allergies effectively. The lungs function best when they are well-hydrated, which means that you need to be well-hydrated. In fact, dehydration alone can trigger an asthma attack. Make sure that the water you're guzzling, however, is pure and clean. You might want to purchase spring water for your drinking needs and use tap water for cooking, cleaning, and bathing. A water filter is a good idea, too. Multi-Pure makes an excellent one (see Appendix B for a distributor).

Food allergies

Food allergies are another culprit in asthmatic and allergic symptoms. In fact, some researchers and practitioners feel that they are *the* culprit, and that identifying and eliminating all foods to which you are allergic can effectively clear up asthma and/or allergy symptoms. A Chinese medical doctor, kinesiologist, or allergist can help you determine whether or not you have allergies to particular foods, which, of course, should be avoided. Another way to approach this is to eliminate suspected food groups from your diet one at a time; then keep a diary or record to see whether this helps or not. Once you pin down a general food group such as dairy or nuts, you can then experiment with adding back individual foods to see if your allergies are more specific. Another method, which is more severe, is to undertake a fast (under the supervision of a health care provider), then add back food groups one at a time and see if any cause you problems. Personally, I favor a less severe approach, but this last method works for many people.

Dairy products

Often practitioners recommend that people who suffer from asthma and allergies avoid dairy products. When I was first starting to get my asthma under control, I cut back considerably on my dairy consumption, but I have since added it back with no negative consequences. Milk that has acidophilus cultures added to it is far easier to digest than plain milk. Raw milk is also easier to digest since the enzymes and microorganisms that help us to assimilate dairy products are not killed by pasteurization. Of course, a small risk of acquiring some type of infection from raw milk exists, but most locales where raw milk is sold have very strict requirements that guarantee the safety of the product. I personally think it is important to eat food that possesses friendly bacteria, which aid in our digestion, recent *E. coli* scares notwithstanding.

Alcohol

Alcohol, which dries out both the intestines and the lungs, is best drunk in moderation or avoided entirely if your asthma is severe. Wine can be particularly troublesome to those who have allergies and asthma, due to the sulfites and tannins that are present. If you drink beer, you should choose brands that are brewed naturally and not chemically fermented. This means selecting imported or microbrew beers. Most commercial American beers are loaded with tons of chemicals to cut down on the brewing time, make it foamy, cut back on the foaminess, etc., etc. They fall into the "chemicals in a can" category.

Caffeine

Caffeinated drinks are a somewhat debatable choice of beverages. Many people find that coffee and tea do no harm, and in fact, the structure of the caffeine molecule is similar in structure to the anti-asthmatic drug, theophylline. Some practitioners even recommend a couple of cups of strong coffee or a chocolate bar as an emergency measure for an asthma attack if nothing else is available. If you brew your own coffee at home, finding organic beans would be well worth the trouble since inorganic coffee is one of the most heavily sprayed crops in the world. Likewise, if you drink decaf, try to find a variety that uses water rather than chemicals to extract the caffeine. Most people do not experience constipation from drinking either coffee or tea (in fact, just the opposite), but if you are like me, and the constituents dry out your colon and slow down your digestion, you would be better off not drinking it. Anything that interferes with healthy and efficient digestion should be eliminated.

Meals

You should pay attention to the rhythm of your eating patterns, too. Letting yourself get really hungry or starving is not a good idea (never skip a meal!); neither is eating too much so that you're uncomfortably full. If your stomach is too full, it can press up against the lungs, reducing your lung volume. In addition, when you eat too much at one time, your digestion is less efficient and this can add toxic by-products to your system, with resulting wheezing and bronchiole constriction. You should eat several small meals a day if at all possible (this might also give you the nice side benefit of helping with weight loss), and definitely try not to eat a big meal right before retiring.

You should also make sure that your diet includes lots of fresh fruits, vegetables, grains, and beans. Meat is not a big problem, but it's better not to eat too much of it. Meat is more difficult to digest than vegetarian fare, can make your colon sluggish, and it creates an unfavorable acidity to your body chemistry. I eat meat, however, including red meat, and don't find it to be a problem, as long as I don't overdo it. Some health practitioners recommend that people with asthma or allergies eat shellfish sparingly or not at all as it contains the highest levels of histamine of any food.

Food combining

Food combining is another technique that many people find helpful in promoting health digestion. This method recommends that you eat proteins and starches separately, the theory being that these two substances require very different digestive enzymes in order to be broken down and assimilated. If you're suffering from a lot of bloating, gas, and intestinal discomfort, it might be worth a try. Vegetables and most fruits can be eaten with either starches or proteins, though acidic fruits such as citrus are consumed only with proteins and some nutritionists feel that fruit is best consumed by itself, particularly melons.

This regimen is not necessarily easy to follow in this society, however, where we have structured our eating habits to include all major food groups in one meal. Meat sandwiches and hamburgers, meat and potatoes, pasta dishes with meat or cheese sauces, fish served with rice, bread with a nonvegetarian meal…all these combinations put proteins and starches together in the same serving. Adhering to this system can require a lot of planning and ingenuity, especially when eating out. Apparently rice and beans are an exception to this regimen; they can be eaten together with no problem. And some proponents of this system feel that fish and rice can be eaten together with no undesirable effects.

Chinese medicine

Chinese medicine may add other considerations to the diet and food picture, since different foods are classified as "hot" or "cold" or drying or moisturizing. If you are seeing a Chinese medical doctor, he or she might have dietary recommendations to suggest. Currently, my acupuncturist is advising that I avoid spicy food, which is hot and drying, since my kidneys have been "dry" and "hot." I should also not drink alcohol while this is a problem. Instead, I should be eating juicy, moisturizing foods such as pears and melons and drinking fresh fruit and vegetable juices.

Diets

In planning your diet, beware of fad or cult diets. These diets pop up all the time and often miraculous claims are made for their effectiveness in curing all kinds of problems; but I would regard any such diet with suspicion. Any extremely restrictive or peculiar diet should be run by your health practitioner first, including a macrobiotic diet. I know that many people have been helped by a macrobiotic diet, but it is restrictive enough that I think it should only be undertaken with a great deal of knowledge and planning.

I have read and heard about many astonishing cures attained through particular diets, so I believe healing through nutrition can be very powerful. I also think that our bodies possess a great deal of their own wisdom, so if a particular diet is bringing you relief or dealing effectively with your symptoms, then you should listen to your body. But use common sense. And do check with your health practitioner before embarking on anything particularly exotic.

Enzymes

Enzymes are another hotly promoted remedy at this time, but I have to say that I am unconvinced of their value. Call me a Luddite if you will, but I think that enzymes are too potent and the full spectrum of their activity is too poorly understood at this time to start ingesting large supplemental quantities. My background is in genetics and molecular biology, and I know for a fact that the same enzymes have different actions in different tissues and organs. Enzymes fall into the same category as pharmaceutical drugs in my opinion. Until we have thoroughly characterized all the effects and pathways that an enzyme might possess or be a part of, I think we are much better off getting our enzymes from food.

Obtaining plenty of active digestive enzymes from our diet is one reason why I think it's important to drink fresh juices that haven't been pasteurized, and why I think raw milk is good for us. I am also tentatively in favor of trying some of the friendly bacterial solutions on the market to improve digestion, though I am still waiting for all the data to come in before jumping in with both feet. Ingesting acidophilus in milk, yogurt, buttermilk, or supplement form seems clearly harmless and beneficial and has been in practice for a long time.

Unless, however, you possess some genetic disease that makes it impossible for you to create or utilize certain necessary enzymes, or you've had your gall bladder or some other organ removed, I would not recommend taking enzymes as dietary supplements. Of course, if your health care practitioner recommends that you take them, you have had good results from taking them, and you feel that ingesting them is clearly helpful and not harmful, then by all means, follow the advice of your health care provider. But to anyone else, I would advise caution.

In summary, use good sense. Follow dietary guidelines that are healthy under any circumstances: buy organic, avoid artificial ingredients, eat plenty of fresh fruits, vegetables, and grains, use pure, cold-pressed oils, drink lots of clean water, and eat several small meals throughout the day. And above all, appreciate and enjoy your food. One of the most odious developments of the current modern era is the idea that it's okay for breakfast to consist of some packaged item that you gobble down as you run out the door. Food is meant to nourish us in all kinds of ways, and other creatures give their lives so that we can sustain ourselves. Treat your body and your food with reverence and respect, and you'll reap many rewards besides just improving your asthma or allergies.

CHIROPRACTIC AND OSTEOPATHY

Chiropractic medicine involves manipulation of the spine and other structures of the skeletal system, whereas osteopathic medicine involves a combination of allopathic healing techniques, such as prescribing drugs, as well as manipulation. Apparently, osteopaths have leaned more toward allopathic methods of healing over the last few years because of insurance considerations and societal biases. But many osteopaths are still excellent sources for spinal manipulation.

The quack factor

Many people regard chiropractors as quacks. The field of allopathic medicine in particular has traditionally maintained an antagonistic stance towards this discipline. And because the field is not as regulated as some would like, critics have charged that the quality of chiropractors is so uneven as to be dangerous. However, while it is true the quality of chiropractors varies, so does the quality of medical doctors. When I worked a year in a hospital as a pulmonary functions technician, what I saw was enough to make me wish fervently that I would never, ever end up in a hospital. In fact, over a hundred thousand deaths a year are attributed to iatrogenic causes, meaning, they happened *because* the person was in the hospital. Unfortunately, many medical doctors are prejudiced and others are simply monopolists: they don't want to share the field of medicine with other disciplines. Others, of course, are intelligent, insightful, helpful, well-trained practitioners. But so are many chiropractors.

The fact is, many, many studies have documented the success of spinal manipulation in the treatment of back pain. People spend less time in bed, take fewer medications, experience less pain, and miss fewer days of work when they receive spinal manipulation for back problems as opposed to those who don't. Allopathic solutions to back pain involve heavy duty drugs that impair function and productivity, such as muscle relaxers and pain meds, bed rest (now recognized to be of debatable value), and surgery.

Because I viewed chiropractors with suspicion in the seventies, I avoided going to see a chiropractor after a very bad cross-country ski accident. I spent the next two years in a tremendous amount of pain. I tried taking muscle relaxants for awhile and hated them since all I felt like doing was sleeping. I had a job and the two were mutually incompatible. Finally, out of nothing but sheer desperation, I went to see a chiropractor, and the relief I received from the first visit was blissfully instantaneous: My pain went away immediately and I went white water rafting that weekend.

Since then, I haven't experienced anything so dramatic from my visits to a chiropractor, but I have become quite a fan. Of course, there are charlatans in the field. I know of one chiropractor who has his whole practice set up to process as many patients as possible and he is a very wealthy man. (Of course, I also know of physicians who have the same set-up.) I would try to find someone with more modest financial aspirations.

I would also view with suspicion any who want to expose your body to lots and lots of x-rays. I would resist buying a million vitamins or supplements from a chiropractor, and I would definitely urge you not to feel obligated to buy the special pillow or the device that supposedly stretches your neck out or any of those apparati. If you really want the pillow, then fine, but an effective chiropractor doesn't need all that paraphernalia. A good chiropractic treatment is a very straightforward affair.

Okay, this all sounds very interesting, you say; but what does it have to do with asthma? Legally, chiropractors cannot claim to treat anything but back problems and associated pain. But in fact, chiropractic and osteopathic manipulation can do much more than that. They just can't advertise this information. And frankly, I would also be leery of a chiropractor who asserts that absolutely everything can be cured by spinal manipulation and only spinal manipulation. But it does have a much wider application than simply back pain.

Method of action in treating asthma

The reason chiropractic medicine can help a wide variety of ailments is due to the way our spine is structured with respect to our circulatory and neurological system. Our spine consists of several hollow chunky bones called vertebrae. They stack up one on top of the other. Inside our vertebrae run arteries and blood vessels, in addition to nerve fibers. On the sides of our spine are gaps between the places where the vertebrae fit together so that blood vessels and nerve fibers can pass from the interior of our spine to all the organs and systems of the body, connecting them to our brain. As we all know, the brain is the command center for the body, and it's critical that information flow freely to and from our organs and brains.

What do you think would happen when one or more of the vertebrae slipped out of the proper position and the vertebrae now mashed down on the blood vessels or nerves running from the spine and brain to the respective organ? That organ wouldn't function so well, would it? It would either be deprived of the blood it needs to both oxygenate and cleanse the organ, and/or the neurological information going between that organ and the brain would be impaired. Either way, the organ function would be compromised. For this reason, when the vertebrae that cup the vessels and nerve fibers servicing the lungs are improperly situated, asthma can result. Edgar Cayce, the well-known trance healer, was an enthusiastic supporter of osteopathic manipulations for asthma. And my current chiropractor tells me that he's adjusted the spines of asthmatic children and watched their breathing ease up right away. He didn't, of course, *claim* that the adjustment relieved the asthma. He merely noted it as an intriguing coincidence.

Recently, through a combination of massage and chiropractic manipulation, a vertebra in my upper back that had been dislodged for at least fourteen years was successfully realigned. Not only is it wonderful not to suffer that constant, niggling pain, I noticed that my lung volume has increased substantially. In addition to the effect described above, I realized that whenever I took a deep breath before this, it would hurt the musculature of my back, my neck, and my chest. So I had just gotten into the unconscious habit of suppressing deep breaths. This, then, is another way that chiropractic or osteopathic adjustments can help asthma: through the relief of constrictive muscle pain.

<u>Finding a practitioner</u>

As with all healers, get a recommendation from someone you know and trust when seeking a chiropractor or osteopath. Some are definitely better than others, some are less expensive than others, and some are less likely to pressure you to come in according to some schedule you don't want to follow than others. Keep in mind that whatever put your spine out in the first place could have taken years; or it might have been years since you dislodged it and the muscles and surrounding ligaments, etc., have all adjusted to this new position. It's unlikely that you will experience immediate relief, though that can happen. I know this firsthand. But don't feel discouraged or blame the practitioner if you don't see God on your first visit. As with many holistic treatments, several visits will no doubt prove necessary.

Also, remember that your skeletal structure is all connected, so it's more than likely that your practitioner will adjust all parts of your spine, and possibly even your feet, hips, etc. He or she might also give you a set of exercises, too, to help stretch and strengthen the muscles affected by the adjustment. When your vertebrae go back into their proper position, they'll pull differently on the muscles connected to them than when they were out of position; so the exercises will help to minimize any discomfort and will keep the muscles from pulling the vertebrae back out of place.

If you don't like the first chiropractor or osteopath you see, try another one. You could even call them up beforehand and ask them about what their treatment entails to see if they're the right practitioner for you.

Massage

Seeking concurrent treatment from a massage therapist can greatly increase your chances of success in getting your spine adjusted easily and quickly; so if you can afford both, you should try both. Tense, seized-up muscles can hold or pull vertebrae out of place, making adjustments difficult. Massage can also help ease muscular tension associated with asthma, and it can contribute to your state of relaxation in general, which is helpful, too. Often, your massage therapist will give you some exercises to help in your treatment, too.

Although many people have no doubt experienced improvement in their allergies from chiropractic treatment, it is less clear that this type of treatment is as directly beneficial for these symptoms as it is for asthma. Overall, however, I am an enthusiastic supporter of chiropractic medicine, and I think it has a lot to offer in the treatment of a number of ailments. Just be sure to choose your healer wisely and give him or her the time he needs to actually get something done. In combination with other treatment options, spinal manipulation can be extremely effective in the management of asthma.

BREATHING AND EXERCISE

Most of us have encountered—to our horror and dismay—the old-fashioned asthmatic child of movies, print media, and television: the neurotic, wimpy, inhaler-clutching dweeb. Because exercise can induce an asthmatic episode, this caricature, sadly enough, contains some truth; and for a long time, both asthmatic children and adults were cautioned not to overexert themselves. Fortunately, high profile athletes who suffer from asthma, such as Jackie Joyner Kersey, have helped to dispel this stereotype; it is now universally recognized that regular exercise helps keep asthma under control. Unfortunately, the solution as presented in the media is simply to haul around one of those inhalers, use a peak-flow meter every day, and take your meds. Then, according to current dogma, everything will be hunky dory. In my experience, though, and perhaps yours as well, it isn't that simple.

As I mentioned in the first chapter, I think it's likely that regular use of an inhaler over time, no matter what kind it is, can set you up for long term rebound effects. In fact, I believe using an inhaler regularly for my exercise-induced asthma is a large part of what got me into trouble with chronic, recurrent episodes later in my life. Instead, I recommend using homeopathic tablets, acupressure points, breathing techniques, and judicious exercising patterns—along with, of course, your ongoing treatment program.

Breathing effectively

Many people who suffer from asthma breathe improperly, in ways that make our asthma worse. We breathe from the top of our lungs, using our chest muscles, and we hyperventilate and breathe shallowly. What we need to do is exactly the opposite.

Effective breathing involves using your diaphragm to draw in your breath. Your diaphragm is a muscular partition that separates the chest and abdominal cavities, and for all intents and purposes in learning how to breathe properly, you can think of it as located in the same general area as your stomach. When you breathe, you should use your diaphragm, inflating it down and outwards; then let the breath travel up and gradually involve the upper reaches of your lungs. Then let it go. You might practice by placing a hand on your stomach when you inhale, pushing out your hand with your diaphragm. You could even imagine a balloon expanding first in your stomach, then in your lungs. You should breathe deeply, slowly, and regularly. Also, be sure to exhale as thoroughly as you can, completely emptying your lungs of air.

For awhile, you should breathe mindfully, perhaps combining breath work with your meditation or relaxation technique. It will take awhile to have this style of breathing come as second nature, but every time you notice yourself breathing shallowly and from the top of your lungs, revert consciously back to diaphragmatic breathing.

Breathing this way will not only improve your asthma, it will deliver more oxygen to all systems of your body, including your brain, which will make you less anxious. It will put less strain on your upper back muscles, which can get very, very sore from straining to breathe. It might also improve your digestion, which is important to keep healthy if you suffer from asthma.

Some people might find that they can benefit most from breath work as taught by a practitioner. If you live in an urban area or locality where alternative health care is popular, you might be able to locate a healer who specializes specifically in breathwork. Some massage therapists include breath work in their repertoire of techniques. Another activity to try is singing or chanting lessons. Singers have to breathe properly or they can't perform well. Another possibility is to take up some sort of wind instrument, like the flute or trumpet. Not only will singing or playing a wind instrument teach you to breathe properly, it can help distract you from your asthma and relax you overall. The vibratory aspects of singing or playing an instrument are generally very healthful as well. Acting lessons or speaking classes often also involve teaching students to breathe effectively, too, so they might be worth a try.

Exercise

An exercise plan is an extremely important part of any asthma management program. Even though you might find that aerobic exercise in particular causes you to wheeze, it's a good idea to continue to pursue exercise. Swimming is often recommended for asthmatics, as it is a gentle form of exercise and involves inhaling water vapor as you swim, which is beneficial for the lungs. Walking, of course, is an excellent activity and shouldn't prompt any type of asthmatic reaction, unless you're out of shape and/or struggling up a very steep hill. Bicycling is my favorite exercise, and though I used to start wheezing when I charged up a hill, I don't anymore. Running is fine if your joints can handle it, dance is terrific, as are any kind of racket sports—in fact, just about any kind of aerobic exercise is good for you overall and in the long term. The more you are able to utilize your full lung volume during exercise without suffering any negative consequences, the healthier your lungs will be, and the less likely you are to experience nonexercise-induced asthma.

Of course, as with any exercise program, be sensible, not macho. If you're out of shape or very asthmatic, start slowly and gently. Don't burden yourself with unrealistic goals that you're going to end up abandoning. I'll never forget the time my husband and I visited the Hoh National Park in Washington state. As we perused the map of the park, we overheard a young woman dressed in loafers and a faux-fur fashion parka saying to her partner: "Why don't we just hike up to the top of Mt. Olympus and back?

It's only thirty-six miles round trip. If we go nine miles an hour, it'll only be four hours." As the possibility of this young lass smoking up the flanks of Mt. Olympus, bounding like Wonder Woman through twenty foot snow drifts seemed unlikely, we were relieved when her companion responded, "Maybe *you* can hike nine miles an hour, but I can't." Later, we saw them on the mile-and-a-half nature trail, as happy as they could be. They enjoyed a nice walk and no one died in the snow.

The main thing is to be persistent. Pick something you really think you'll enjoy and stick with it. If you're over fifty or feeling cautious, check your program out with your health care provider. You might want to start with walking and/or swimming, then move on to more vigorous exercise. One type of exercise you should to be careful with, however, is in the area of winter sports. Inhaling very cold air, especially if you're breathing hard, can often trigger an attack. Once you've built up your stamina and resistance, however, you might find that you don't have this problem.

This is the method I developed to handle my exercise-induced asthma (although, as I've said, I no longer experience this type of episode): If I find myself wheezing, I ease up the intensity of my activity right away, but I don't stop. If I'm biking up a steep hill, I'll get off my bike and walk. If I'm running, I slow down to a lazy jog. If I'm walking hard, I reduce my pace. I make sure that I'm breathing from my diaphragm and I consciously make my breathing as slow and deep as I can. Then I take a homeopathic tablet. If my hands are free, I'll stimulate the acupressure points described in Appendix A for a few minutes. I make sure I'm well hydrated, too. And then, if my breathing still hasn't gotten any better, I'll use my inhaler as a last resort.

The more you treat your lungs to aerobic activity without triggering an asthmatic episode, the more you'll be able handle the next time you exercise. Exercising represents a highly positive feedback loop, where the more you do, the more you can do. Believe me, over time, your lungs will love you for it. And so will the rest of your body. Just take it easy and take your time building up to vigorous activity.

Proper breathing and exercise alone will probably not manage your asthma entirely, but they are very important components to any strategy you employ. In fact, you should not leave them out, no matter what else you're doing. The combination of good breathing technique and regular exercise will strengthen your lungs, keep them supple, and desensitize them to irritants. And as an added bonus, you will enjoy greater energy, strength, and psychological well-being.

MISCELLANEOUS CONSIDERATIONS

There are a few other useful tactics to employ in managing your health that I would like to mention in this chapter. Another book that you might find helpful in dealing with your asthma and allergies is my previous title, THE NATURAL REMEDIES FOR COMMON AILMENTS HANDBOOK, which gives drug-free alternatives to everyday health problems so that you don't have to use over-the-counter drugs. Keeping the number of pharmaceutical drugs you use to a minimum will help you to manage your asthma by keeping your organs healthy and minimizing your exposure to toxins and side-effects.

Supplements

Supplements are big business these days and some of them definitely fall into the category of snake oil. Others, however, are quite helpful. And of course, some are useful to some people and not to others. Not everyone is necessarily going to benefit from the same supplement; it depends on your genetic makeup, the environment you live in, your diet, your mental/emotional state, your history, and many other factors. Therefore, once again I'm going to exhort you to take responsibility for your own health and use your own judgment in determining which, if any, supplements you should use. I personally am always suspicious of any supplements that are touted as miracle cures, or sold by people who are part of some kind of pyramid selling scheme.

Glandulars

When I first saw an acupuncturist for my asthma, the practitioner had me take a type of supplement known as glandulars. In essence, these supplements are ground-up organs from an animal, usually a cow. I took ground-up cow's lung and ground-up cow's uterus (since my practitioner detected a weakness in that organ as well). Glandulars exist for just about every organ in the human body. After I had received several months' worth of treatment, he discontinued the glandulars.

Since I was also receiving acupuncture treatments, taking herbs, and changing my diet, it's difficult for me to ascertain whether the glandulars were helpful. I know they didn't hurt and my acupuncturist seemed to think they were working, so, it seems to me a perfectly harmless, potentially beneficial thing to try. You can, however, pursue a successful regimen without including them, in my opinion.

Blue-green algae

Blue-green algae is a very trendy supplement right now, and it is one of those extolled as a miracle cure for absolutely everything under the sun. It is a nutrient-rich supplement, and all the ingredients together supposedly oxygenate the body, which is certainly desirable. Taking some is surely helpful in a general way for asthma and allergies, but I don't know that it lives up to much of its sensationalistic billing. As blue-green algae is so hot right now, obtaining it should be easy. Your local health food store probably carries it, or you can check Appendix B for a supplier.

Tonics

As I mentioned in the chapter on Western herbs, herbal tonics are a safe and healthful supplement to any health program, particularly ones involving asthma and allergies. Try tinctures, teas, freeze-dried extracts, tablets or capsules made with red clover, stinging nettles, Astralagus, or Siberian ginseng.

Minerals

Another supplement making the rounds these days is colloidal minerals. Apparently, minerals in colloidal form are the most easily absorbed by the body. So, you're actually retaining what you're swallowing. Most colloidal mineral solutions contain anywhere from thirty to ninety (or more!) minerals, although colloidal silver is often sold on its own for various purposes.

The theory behind taking extensive mineral supplements is a sound one, in my view. Human beings are extremely complex biological organisms. We possess hundreds of thousands of genes, countless proteins and enzymes, and all kinds of other biological molecules. Enzymes, the expediters of molecular tasks, work in this way: They have two (at least) shapes that they can assume. When they are in one configuration, they're inert; they don't interact with anything. When they occupy another configuration, they zoot over to their active site and clomp on and perform a kind of molecular magic. They cause a chemical reaction to take place in lightning speed and at biologically safe temperatures that would ordinarily require two centuries or several thousand degrees of heat. Many enzymes are activated by the placement of an elemental ion in their structure, such as zinc or magnesium. If the zinc or magnesium isn't available, the enzyme can't change its shape into the active one, and therefore, it can't catalyze the reaction it would normally catalyze. So the work doesn't get done.

Over the centuries, our current farming methods have leached the micronutrients from the soil. Plants take up minerals for their enzymes in just the same way that we use them. After awhile, unless these micronutrients are replaced, they no longer exist in the soil. Annual flooding from undammed rivers used to replace the minerals, as does snow melt coming out of the mountains. But now flooding rarely, if ever takes place. And most of the places where our food crops are grown don't receive snow melt. Most farmers add fertilizers to the soil that contain only a handful of the original nutrients (such as nitrogen, phosphorus, and potassium). This is why organic fertilizers are often superior to inorganic ones: they contain a larger number of nutrients. But, since these animals who produce the fertilizer are often eating from the same nutrient-poor crop areas as we are, they are deficient as well.

It would be difficult for a body to operate at its optimum level if it lacked any of its important enzymes' active configurations. Moreover, since it is highly likely that the shape of our genetic regulatory proteins determine which genes are read, even the production of certain necessary biomolecules could depend on maintaining all the essential nutrients in our bodies. I have been taking colloidal minerals for several weeks now, and I find that I have more energy, feel more relaxed, and my asthma seems to have improved even more. You can often buy colloidal mineral supplements at your health food store (be forewarned: they're pricey!), or you can order them through any number of catalogs that sell vitamins. Check Appendix B for a source.

It's possible, of course, that some people might have a sensitivity to any one of the micronutrients included in these colloidal mixes; so if you experience any negative effects after you start taking them, discontinue their use.

An alternative to taking mineral supplements is to use Celtic sea salt. This salt comes directly from the nutrient-rich ocean and is not processed in such a way that many of the micronutrients are lost. It's wet when you receive or buy it, and it's a lovely, pearly grayish color. It turns whiter as it dries. Check to see if your favorite health food store carries it, or order Celtic Sea Saltô from the Grain & Salt Society (see Appendix B). They carry a particularly fine product.

Vitamins

Many practitioners feel that vitamin therapy can make a big difference in managing asthma and allergies. In his book, THE COMPLETE MANUAL OF NATURAL ALLERGY CONTROL, Dr. David Williams recommends taking 2000 to 5000 mg of vitamin C a day (making sure also to obtain enough calcium, which vitamin C leaches from the body), 500 to 1500 mg of bioflavanoids (spread throughout the day and taken at the same time as the vitamin C), a daily B vitamin supplement that contains as least 50 mg. of each B vitamin (or take 2 heaping tablespoons of nutritional yeast each day), 200 to 500 mg of pantothenic acid per day, 200 to 500 units of vitamin E daily, in addition to 10,000 units of vitamin A.

Bee pollen and honey

Bee pollen is another supplement widely recommended for help with allergies. I've taken it, with no noticeable results, but others have found relief with it. You should be aware of the fact, though, that taking bee pollen has sent certain sensitive individuals into severe allergic reactions. So, if you decide to try it, you might want to start out taking a very, very small dose and build up. And have your emergency measures in place when you do so.

A safer alternative is simply eating a couple of teaspoons of local honey everyday, as the pollen in honey is less concentrated. Spread it on bread, take it straight, or add it to your tea or yogurt—whatever. Choose a honey that is local, though, since it will have the pollens you're exposed to; and choose one that has honey derived from as many sources as possible, too (select wildflower honey, for example, as opposed to that obtained strictly from orange blossoms or clover). Farmer's markets, roadside stands, and health food stores are good sources for local honey.

<u>Natural inhalers</u>

Several natural inhalers exist to try, in place of the chemical-based ones. One is based on Edgar Cayce remedies, and it is sold by The Heritage Store under the name of Inspirol. To be honest, I've tried it and not found it to help all that much; but I am a big admirer of Edgar Cayce, so it might be that you would find that it works for you. It might be worth a try, as it's not all that expensive.

An Edgar Cayce product that I have found to be useful along these lines, though, is the Heritage Store's Scarmassage ointment, which is designed to make scars go away (which, in fact, it does, if you are very persistent).

Perhaps it is primarily the camphor that is so helpful. It doesn't exactly make me feel like Isabella Rosselini, but I have found that dabbing some on my wrists and inhaling the fumes will often ease tightness in my chest and any wheezing I might be experiencing. Again, it's not that expensive, and it also works for scars, so you might want to check it out. Information for The Heritage Store is listed in Appendix B.

White Flower Balm, which is an Oriental remedy for muscle aches and pains, is another a volatile oil that can help ease wheezing, tightness in the chest, and stuffed-up sinuses. Bring a big pot of water to a boil, sprinkle in a few drops of the oil, put a towel over your head and then lean over the pot, inhaling the steam. Take the pot off the flame first, of course, to avoid setting your towel and hair on fire. Appendix B gives a mail-order source for White Flower Balm.

I have also found the essential oils of pine, eucalyptus, and even peppermint or spearmint to be helpful in opening up my lungs and sinuses. Pine is known for its expectorant qualities, whereas eucalyptus is a decongestant. Mint is not really known for either of these properties, but the freshness and volatility of the substances seem to do something for opening up clogged passageways. Use these essential oils in the same way that you would use the White Flower Balm; look for them at your health food store.

A nice combination remedy for breathing the vapor is composed of the essential oils of thyme, eucalyptus, rosemary, and ginger. Sprinkle a few drops into the water you'll be heating up and inhaling as described above.

There are also essential oil lamps that you can buy which will release the volatiles into the air of the room you're in. Or, you can take a pan full of water and drops of these oils and place it on your radiator or woodstove.

I would like to mention Euphorbium again in this context, an herbal nasal spray that is extremely effective for sinuses, somewhat effective for asthma, and which has no rebound effects. It not only opens up stuffed-up passageways, it clears them of mucus, and it's easy to use. You can obtain this product from Shanah Azee, listed in Appendix B.

If the climate you're living in is extremely dry (like summers in Arizona or winters in the Northeast), it would help to hydrate your lungs. Besides drinking plenty of water, you can purchase one of those plant misters and spray it in your face while you breathe for a few minutes. Replace the mister frequently so that mold doesn't build up in any of the working parts. In fact, it is recommended that you not use a humidifier as they are notorious for harboring mold; but a vaporizer should be okay since it steams the water. The high heat keeps it less moldy.

The nasal douche

Doesn't sound appealing, does it? Well, it's not, really. But the aftermath can be delightful. First, obtain some good sea salt that's not all dried out (like the Celtic Sea Saltô mentioned above). Gather up some hydrogen peroxide, a dropper, mortar and pestle, and one of those rubber bulbs (like the ones used to irrigate kids' ears with).

Take a small pinch of salt and grind it up with the mortar and pestle. Then add a few ounces of water, so that the mixture tastes like sea water (too concentrated a solution will dry out your sinuses; too dilute won't work as well). Using the dropper, add 5 to 10 drops of hydrogen peroxide to the salt and water mixture, stir it well with the pestle, and then draw up some of the liquid with the rubber bulb. Making sure you have a towel or some tissues handy, tilt your head back a little, place the tip of the bulb in either nostril, and squeeze gently. Saltwater will go rushing into your sinus cavities, down the back of your throat, and all over the front of your face. This is where the towel or tissues come in handy. Repeat two or three times for each nostril, then blow your nose.

While you're engaged in this procedure, you're probably not having the time of your life. In fact, it will probably feel weird. But afterwards! Ah . . . afterwards, it feels great! Your sinuses are all cleaned out of pollen and all kinds of other stuff you don't necessarily want in there, and they feel refreshed and clear. Do this once or twice a day if you're really suffering. Another good thing to do during allergy season is to get in the shower and just let the water run all over your face. This is particularly helpful for itchy eyes as well as sinuses.

<u>Eye drops</u>

Herbal eye drops can help a great deal if your allergies are making you feel like you want to claw your eyes out from itchiness and irritation. Similasan makes a very nice herbal eye drop, and you can often find them at your health food store. You can also order them through Home Health (listed in Appendix B).

As you can see, there are many, many options to managing your asthma and allergies. Most of them are highly superior to pharmaceutical options, in my view, not only in their absence of side-effects but in their effectiveness, too. You'll be much better off if you can find and implement a successful holistic strategy before you end up on steroids, since once you start taking something like prednisone, you alter your physiology significantly. This then becomes another problem that you have to address in your treatment. If you are currently on steroids, however, you can still benefit from alternative methods, and you can, in fact, improve so much that you can stop taking them. I would like to stress once again, however, that you should not just stop taking any medication that you are currently using. You should work closely with a health care practitioner who can help ease you off any medication you'd like to quit.

The one pharmaceutical drug that I still continue to take is an antihistamine during the worst of our pollen season. But, I now take these drugs only a few weeks out of the year instead of six months out of the year. And I'm hoping that eventually, I won't have to take them at all. I don't notice many tangible side-effects, but I know that I'm not doing my liver or heart any favors by taking them. However, I am not using any medication whatsoever to manage my asthma on a daily basis—only an occasional use of an inhaler for emergencies, usually fewer than four times a year. I manage my asthma year round with a combination of the methods I've described here. And I was in very bad shape to begin with.

Before I end the discussion, I would like to make one other observation. The rise in asthma (and allergies) is clearly related to conditions in our environment. As I mentioned in Chapter 1, I think this is due to a combination of factors, from pollution to stress to wishful magical thinking in the form of false magic bullets. Our society has gotten off track with the introduction of concepts like "The Bottom Line." The pursuit of health and happiness has become one of its casualties. If we are to believe what the media projects, life has now become nothing more than trying to figure out how to make the most money, how to spend the most money, and how to keep our jobs, our benefits, our houses, and our cars.

The pace of life in striving to meet the requirements of this "bottom line" existence has accelerated to an extremely unhealthy, even insane tempo. Asthma is only one symptom of a global society proceeding blithely down a path of truly mindless production and consumption, supporting unhealthy values. We see it in the increase of all types of chronic diseases, from cancer, to heart disease, to depression. We see it in the breakdown of our families and communities; we see it in increased poverty and violence.

We have it in our power to reject false values. We can resist downsizing of our emotional and spiritual lives even if we can't fight the downsizing in our places of work.

We can reimbue our lives with healthy values such as making plenty of time to spend with our partners and children, our extended families and our friends. It is *not* frivolous or unproductive to slow down and enjoy a leisurely meal, a walk, or a good book; in fact, these things are essential to our mental and physical health. We can opt for greater free time over earning more money, develop our hidden talents, and fulfill some of our most cherished private dreams. We can make sacrifices in our possessions and economic standard of living and reap huge benefits in our emotional, psychological, and spiritual well-being.

As near-death expert P. M. H. Atwater commented in a lecture I attended recently, those who have crossed over to the other side and then come back never say, "I wish I'd made more money," or "I wish I'd worked harder to get that promotion." They invariably say, "I wish I'd spent more time with my kids," or "I wish I'd been more loving." Health is a vastly complex, interconnected, and powerful state of being. Let's seize it with both hands; and let's live our lives to their absolute fullest.

Appendix A

Acupressure Points

Asthma Points

Locate your sternum, or breastbone, in the center of your chest. The ribs attach here and form little sockets, or depressions, inbetween each rib. Start at the top, underneath your collar bone, and work your way down, digging your index fingers into each depression for 30 seconds to several minutes. Be sure that your fingers are nestled up against your sternum and inbetween the ribs. Spend the most time on the ones that seem to be the most tender. Once you get down about five or six ribs, you can stop. If there are one or two spots that seem to be the most effective in easing up your breathing, concentrate on those. It might sound counter-intuitive to press on any part of your chest when you're having trouble breathing, but this can often ease up your breathing immediately.

Another set of points is located about an inch or so below your collar bone. Find it by clasping the tendon that leads from your arm to your chest. Your fingers will be tucked into your armpit and your thumbs should be resting on the acupressure spot. Poke around a little bit to find a sore place; if you discover one, dig your thumbs in there, or use your fingers. Apply pressure for several minutes.

One final point to try is the one right inside the depression formed inbetween your collarbones at the base of your throat and the top of your breastbone. Press your finger at the bottom of that little dip in the bone, inside the concavity. As always, search for a tender spot, which is usually the point you're looking for.

Allergy Points

These points are pretty easy to locate. The first ones are found on either side of your nose, right on either side of your nostrils. I find it's easier to use my thumbs than my fingers for these points, but you might prefer using your index fingers. Look for the place where the bone starts to curve in towards your mouth; also look for tender spots. Press diligently.

Another set of points is located below the center of your cheekbones. Nuzzle your thumbs right underneath the cheekbone, right at their center of where they are most rounded; you should find a little socket there. Press relatively hard for a few minutes. You can also just follow along the curve of your cheekbone, from your nose to where your jaw attaches, and press any sore places you find for a few minutes.

Appendix B

Resources

American Association of Naturopathic Physicians
(206) 323-7610
2366 Eastlake Ave., Suite 322
Seattle, WA   98102

BioEnergetics
(800) 334-4043, phone; also (503) 668-7478
Allergy drops, sinus drops, stress drops

Coming Home
(800) 345-3696, phone
(800) 332-0103, fax
Cotton pillows and bedding

Co-op America
(202) 872-5307, phone
1612 K Street NW, Suite 600
Washington, DC   20006
Earth-friendly product directory

Eclectic Institute
(800) 332-4372, phone; also (503) 668-4120
Alfalfa, elecampane, ginkgo, horehound, hyssop, lobelia, marshmallow, mullein, nettles, red clover, Siberian ginseng, Yerba santa

Ellon USA Inc.
(800) 423-2256,phone
(516) 593-9668, fax
English flower remedies

Flower Essence Services
(800) 548-0075, phone
(916) 265-6467, fax
Flower remedies, both English and North American

Flower Essence Society
(800)736-9222, phone
(916)265-0584, fax
E-mail: Info@flowersociety.org
Web site: www.flowersociety.org
Holistic health practitioner database

Garnet Hill
(800) 622-6216, phone
Cotton pillows, bedding, clothing

Grain & Salt Society, Inc.
(800) 867-5800
Celtic Sea Saltô

Hendricksen Natürlich Flooring
(707) 824-0914, phone
P O Box 1677
Sebastopol, CA   95473
Flooring materials

Herb Pharm
(800) 348-4372, phone
(800) 545-7392, fax
Alfalfa, astralagus, elecampane, ginkgo, horehound, hyssop, marshmallow, mullein, nettles, red clover, Siberian ginseng, Yerba santa

The Heritage Store
(800) 862-2923, phone
(800) 329-2292, fax
Blue-green algae, cola syrup, Inspirol, Scarmassage, shampoos, lotions, soaps, etc.

Home Health
(800) 284-9123, phone
(800) 285-8155, fax
Blue-green algae, cola syrup, Similasan eye drops, shampoos, lotions, soaps, cosmetics, etc.

Indiana Botanic Gardens
(219) 947-4040, phone
P O Box 5
Hammond, IN   46325
Lungwort, Irish moss, plus other herbs

Multi-Pure (Ariela Gregorio, distributor)
(800) 201-7108
P O Box 478
Williamsburg, MA   01096
Water filter

Seventh Generation
(800) 456-1177
360 Interlocken Blvd., Suite 300
Broomfield, CO 80021
Cotton bedding, pillows, nontoxic cleaners, housewares

Shanah Azee
(800) 945-0409, phone
(800) 689-6674, fax
E-mail: HealthiMed@aol.com
BHI asthma tablets, Heel (Euphorbium nasal spray) and Shaklee products, astralagus, elecampane, ginkgo, horehound, lobelia, marshmallow, mullein, nettles, red clover, Siberian ginseng, Yerba santa

TransPacific Health Products
(800) 336-9636
White Flower Balm

The Vitamin Shoppe
(800) 223-1216, phone
(800) 852-7153, fax
Vitamins, colloidal minerals

Zia Cosmetics
(800) 334-7546, phone
(415) 543-7694, fax
Skin care products, cosmetics

Appendix C
Summary of Treatments

CHINESE MEDICINE

Needles inserted into points in the body balance organ function and energy pathways of the body.

Herbs are prescribed by a practitioner (may include Ephedra, Astralagus, Ginkgo, Pinellia, Magnolia, Minor Bupleurum, Licorice, Cinnamon, Peony, Ginger, Ophiopogon).

Diet is assessed and often changed.

WESTERN HERBAL REMEDIES

Tonics: Stinging Nettles, Red Clover, Siberian Ginseng
For improved digestion: Yerba Santa, Marshmallow
Expectorants and immune enhancers: Thyme, Mullein, Elecampane,
Other herbs to try: Hyssop, Alfalfa, Lobelia, Lungwort, Irish Moss, Horehound
Balm for chest using essential oils: Into ½ oz almond oil, ½ oz grapeseed oil, put 5 drops thyme, 6 drops eucalyptus, 10 drops rosemary, 14 drops ginger; mix together and apply.
Euphorbium nasal spray
Flower essences address emotional factors

MIND/BODY TECHNIQUES

Visualization
Meditation
Relaxation techniques
Biofeedback

HOMEOPATHY

Combination homeopathic remedies:
  Allergies:
    BioEnergetics' Allergy Drops
    BioEnergetics' Sinus Drops
  Asthma:
    BHI's Asthma Tablets

ENVIRONMENTAL FACTORS

Avoid:
  Mold and dust
  Wall-to-wall carpeting
  Building materials that contain lots of glue
  Paint, stain, copier, and other volatile fumes
  Dry cleaning
  Scented detergents; fabric softeners
  Perfumes, colognes, heavily scented cosmetics and
    toiletries
  Animal dander
  Smoke

Do:

> Keep house dust and pollen-free, dry and clean
> Use hard floor coverings such as tile
> Use natural cleaning products
> Use unscented, people-friendly detergents, cosmetics
> Find a good pillow

EATING HABITS

Avoid:

> Artificial ingredients, additives, preservatives, food colorings
> Foods to which you're allergic
> Sweets, particularly white cane sugar
> Unsaturated fats and oils such as lard, shortening, margarine, palm, cottonseed, and partially hydrogenated soybean oil
> Dairy products
> Alcohol; soft drinks
> Overeating; getting too hungry
> Fad diets

Use:

> Organic and non-processed foods
> Honey, maple syrup, rice syrup, beet sugar
> Extra virgin olive oil, canola oil, peanut oil, sesame oil, butter
> Lots of pure, clean water to drink
> Organic coffee, both caffeinated and decaffeinated
> Foods that contain plenty of fiber, vitamins, and minerals

OSTEOPATHY AND CHIROPRACTIC

Supplement with massage and exercises to strengthen and
stretch muscles
Give it time to work

BREATHING AND EXERCISE

Breathe from your diaphragm
Pursue activities that train you to breathe properly, such
as singing, chanting, playing a wind instrument, or
public speaking
Get plenty of exercise, aerobic and nonaerobic
Use homeopathic tablets and acupressure points to
counteract exercise-induced asthma; use your inhaler
as a last resort

MISCELLANEOUS CONSIDERATIONS

Supplements to try:

Vitamins (daily):

2000 to 5000 mg of vitamin C
500 to 1500 mg of bioflavanoids
B vitamins, 50 mg or more of each B vitamin (or
take 2 heaping Tbs. of nutritional yeast)
200 to 500 mg of pantothenic acid
200 to 800 units of vitamin E
10,000 units of vitamin A

Other supplements:

> Glandulars
> Blue-green algae
> Colloidal minerals
> Quercetin

Natural inhalers:

> Inspirol (from Heritage Store)
> Scarmassage (also from Heritage Store)

> Sprinkle a few drops of the following substances into
> water that you have brought to a boil:
> White flower balm
> Essential oils of pine, eucalyptus, peppermint, or
> spearmint
> Or make mixture of: essential oils of thyme
> eucalyptus, rosemary, and ginger

Use a vaporizer or mister during dry seasons; avoid
humidifiers

Try a nasal douche (see pp. 94–95)

Use herbal eye drops made by Similasan (available from
Home Health)

INDEX

Acidophilus 71–72
Acupressure 18, 21, 99
Acupuncture 10, 14, 16, 17,
    18, 19, 20, 21, 105
Additives 60–62, 107
Adrenal glands 11, 25, 64
Aerobic exercise 83, 84–85
Air pollution 3–4
Alcohol 67, 107
Alfalfa 27, 101, 103, 105
Allergens 1, 7, 55, 56
Allergist 65–66
Allergy drops 101, 106
American Association of
    Naturopathic Physi-
    cians 23, 101
Animals 54–56, 106
Antihistamine 96
Anxiety 28, 82
Aromatherapy 93–94, 109
Artificial ingredients 60–62,
    107
Artificial sweeteners 63
Asthma medication 6
Asthma tablets 104, 106
Astralagus 26, 88, 104, 105

B vitamins 91, 108
Bacteria 66
Bedding 53, 102, 104
Bee pollen 91
Beer 67

BHI 43, 104, 106
BioEnergetics 43, 101, 106
Biofeedback 35, 37, 106
Bioflavanoids 91, 108
Biologic Homeopathic
    Industries 43
Blue-green algae 88, 103, 109
Brain 76–77, 82
Breathing techniques 81–82,
    108
Breathwork 82
Bronchioles 1, 14
Building materials 49–50, 59,
    102, 106, 107
Butter 65

Caffeinated beverages 67–68
Caffeine 67–68
Calcium 91
Camphor 93
Cats 54–56
Cayce, Edgar 8, 76, 92
Celtic sea salt 90–91, 94–95,
    102
Chemicals 49, 50–51, 53, 58,
    59, 67
Chinese medicine 9–21, 65–
    66, 70, 105
Chiropractic 73–79, 108
Chocolate 67–68
Cinnamon 14, 105
Cleaning products 50–51, 107

Clothing 50, 53
Coffee 67–68, 107
Cola syrup 63, 103
Cold air 84
Colloidal minerals 88–89, 90, 109
Cologne 51–53, 106
Colon 11
Coming Home 53, 101
Conditioner 52–53, 61
Corticosteroid inhalers 5–6
Cosmetics 53, 61, 103, 104, 106

Dairy products 66, 71, 107
Del Guidici, Emilio 40
Deodorant 52
Detergents 51, 107
Diaphragm 81
Diaphragmatic breathing 81–82
Diet 60, 66, 68, 70, 70–71, 72, 105, 107
Digestion 11, 105
Dogs 55
Down 53
Drugs 6, 9, 12, 13, 14, 15, 22, 61, 73, 86, 96
Dry cleaning 50, 106
Dust 47–49, 53, 58, 106, 107
Dust mites 47, 49, 53

Earth Rite 50
Eating habits 60–72
Eclectic Institute 101
Eczema 15, 25

Elecampane 26, 101, 103, 104, 105
Electromagnetic fields 3–4, 31
Ellon USA 29, 102
Emotions 28, 30, 31, 36
Endorphins 17
Environment of body 14–15
Enzymes 71–72, 89, 90
Ephedra 14, 27, 105
Essential oils 26, 93, 105, 109
  eucalyptus 26, 93, 105, 109
  ginger 26, 105, 109
  peppermint 93, 109
  pine 93, 109
  rosemary 26, 105, 109
  spearmint 93, 109
  thyme 26, 105, 109
Eucalyptus 26
Euphorbium 25, 94, 104, 105
Exercise 80–85, 108
Exercise program 83–84
Exercise-induced asthma 84–85, 108
Expectorants 24, 26, 105
Eye drops 95, 103, 109

Fabric softeners 51
Fats 64–65, 107
Fiberfill 53
Five Elements 10, 12
Flower Essence Services 29, 102
Flower Essence Society 23, 43, 102
Flower remedies 28–29, 102, 105

Food 13–14
Food allergies 21, 65–66, 107
Food colorings 60–62, 107
Food combining 69
Food diary 66
Freeze-dried extracts 16, 24
Fruits 68, 69, 72

Garnet Hill 53, 102
Genes 31, 89
Genetics 2–3
Ginger 14, 26, 105
Ginkgo 26, 101, 103, 104, 105
Glandulars 87, 109
Grain & Salt Society 91, 102

Hahnemann, Samuel 39–40
Hay fever 18, 21, 24, 25, 43,
    93, 94–95
Headaches 21
Healing crisis 44
Health insurance 19
Health practitioner data-
    base 102
Heart 6, 9, 11, 14, 16, 27
Heel 25, 104
Hendricksen Natürlich
    Flooring 102
Herb Pharm 103
Herbalist 15–16, 22–29
Herbs 10, 12, 14, 15–16, 16,
    21, 22, 22–29, 23, 27, 28,
    29, 105
Heritage Store 92, 103, 109
Histamine 1, 2, 25, 69
Home Health 96, 103, 109

Homeopathy 38–46
    classic 42
    combination 43
    remedies 43, 44–46, 56,
        106, 108
Honey 57, 92
Horehound 27, 101, 103, 104,
    105
Horses 55
Humidifier 94, 109
Hyssop 101, 103, 105

Iatrogenic disease 74
Immune enhancers 25, 26, 105
Immune system 2, 31, 62
Indiana Botanic Gardens 103
Inhalers 108
Inspirol 92, 103, 109
Irish moss 27, 103, 105

Kidneys 11, 64
Kinesiology 16, 65–66

Lesions 5
Licorice 14, 105
Ligaments 77
Liver 6, 11, 64
Lobelia 27, 101, 105
Lungs 1, 5, 6, 11, 12, 76, 81,
    82, 83, 85, 94
Lungwort 103, 105

Ma-huang 14, 27
Magnolia 105
Marshmallow 25, 101, 103,
    104, 105

Massage 78–79, 108
Meals 68–69, 72
Meat 68
Meditation 33, 37, 106
Meridians 10, 17, 18
Milk 71
Mind-body techniques 30–37, 106
Minerals 88–91
Minor Bupleurum 105
Mold 43–44, 48, 49, 94, 106
Moxibustion 10
Mullein 26, 101, 103, 104, 105
Multi-Pure 65, 103
Muscle testing 16
Muscles 77
Musculature 77

National Green Pages 58
Natural inhalers 92–94, 109
Naturopathy 23
Nettles 24, 101, 103, 104
Neuropeptides 31
Nontoxic cleaners 104

Oils 64–65, 72, 107
Ophiopogon 105
Organic foods 62–63
Osteopathy 73–79, 108

Pantothenic acid 91, 108
Peony 14, 105
Perfume 51–53, 106
Pesticides 59
Pets 54–56

Pillows 53–54, 102, 104, 107
Pinellia 105
Pollen 57–58, 107
Pollution 3–4, 97
Prednisone 9, 96
Preservatives 60–62, 107
Processed food 60–62
Proteins 69, 89

Qi 10
Quercetin 25, 109

Red clover 25, 88, 101, 103, 104, 105
Regulatory proteins 31, 90
Relaxation techniques 33, 34, 106
Rhinitis 21
Rice 69
Rosemary 26

Scarmassage 92, 103, 109
Seasonality 12
Seventh Generation 53, 104
Shaklee 50, 104
Shampoo 52–53, 61
Shanah Azee 94, 104
Shellfish 69
Siberian ginseng 25, 88, 101, 103, 104, 105
Side-effects 9
Similasan 95, 109
Sinus drops 43, 101, 106
Sinuses 21, 24, 25, 43, 94–95, 109
Skeletal system 73–79

Skin care products 104
Skin conditions 15
Smoke 57, 106
Soft drinks 63, 107
Spinal manipulation 73–79
Spine 76–77
Spleen 11
Starches 69
Steroids 9–10, 96
Stimulants 24, 27
Stinging nettle 24, 88, 105
Stomach 68
Stress 4, 28, 30, 97
Stress drops 101
Succussion 40
Sugar 63–64, 107
Sulfites 67
Supplements 86–91, 108–109
Sweeteners 63–64, 107
  artificial 63, 64
  honey 64, 107
  maple syrup 64, 107
  rice syrup 64, 107
  sugar 63–64, 107
Sweets 63–64, 107
Swimming 83, 84

Tannins 67
Tea, black 67–68
Teas 15–16, 24
Tension 34
Thyme 105
Tinctures 24
Tonics 24–25, 105
Toxins 4, 6, 7, 60, 86
TransPacific Health Products 104

Triggers 2–3

Urban areas 3–4

Vaporizer 109
Vegetables 68, 69, 72
Vertebrae 76–77, 78
Visualization 30, 32, 35, 37, 106
Vitamin Shoppe 104
Vitamins 91, 108
  vitamin A 91, 108
  vitamin B 91, 108
  vitamin C 91, 108
  vitamin E 91, 108
Walking 83, 84
Water 65, 72, 94, 107
Water filter 65, 103,
Weil, Andrew 24–25
Western herbal medicine 22–29
White Flower Balm 93, 104, 109
Winter sports 84
Wood stoves 57
Wool 49, 53

Yerba santa 25, 101, 103, 104, 105
Yogurt 71

Zia Cosmetics 104

About the Author

Celeste White is a science writer, researcher, and theorist, currently living in Northern California. Winner of the Belyea Botany Prize from Wellesley College, where she graduated a Wellesley Scholar, she also possesses an M.S. in Botany from the University of Massachusetts, where she studied under a University Fellowship. Her first book was THE NATURAL REMEDIES FOR COMMON AILMENTS HANDBOOK.

To obtain additional copies of NATURAL ASTHMA AND ALLERGY MANAGEMENT, check your local book store or health food store, or send your name, address, and daytime telephone number, along with a check or money order for $8.95 plus $2.50 shipping/handling (California residents add 7.25% sales tax) *per book* to:

KESWICK HOUSE
P O Box 992535
Redding, CA   96099-2535

For more information about our press, authors, or other titles, check out our Web site at:

www.snowcrest.net/keswick